TAKE CONTROL OF YOUR ENDOMETRIOSIS

TAKE CONTROL OF YOUR ENDOMETRIOSIS

Help relieve symptoms with simple diet and lifestyle changes

Henrietta Norton

Kyle Books

To any woman with the courage to make a change

First published in Great Britain in 2012 by
Kyle Books
an imprint of Kyle Cathie Limited
23, Howland Street
London W1T 4AY
general.enquiries@kylebooks.com
www.kylebooks.com

ISBN: 978 0 85783 068 5

A CIP catalogue record for this title is available from the British Library

10 9 8 7 6 5 4 3 2 1

Henrietta Norton is hereby identified as the author of this work in accordance with
Section 77 of the Copyright, Designs and Patents Act 1988

Editor: Vicky Orchard
Design: Nicky Collings
Production: Gemma John and Nic Jones

Typeset by Avon DataSet Ltd, Bidford on Avon, Warwickshire

Printed and bound by Martins the Printers Ltd, Berwick upon Tweed

CONTENTS

FOREWORD

Professor Christopher Sutton MA MB BChir FRCOG

Professor of Gynaecological Surgery, Faculty of Health Sciences,
University of Surrey, Guildford, UK.

My first involvement with endometriosis was when I was appointed Consultant Gynaecologist in Guildford with a remit to start a colposcopy service to treat women with abnormal cervical smears with the laser, considered at that time as a revolutionary new treatment. As is so often the case with the NHS no funds were forthcoming to purchase equipment for this new initiative so with the help of some very enthusiastic ladies from Surrey we started the Guildford 'Raise a Laser' Appeal and thanks to the generosity of the local community soon had enough funds to equip a first class colposcopy suite and sufficient money to adapt the laser to act as a precise surgical tool for the treatment of endometriosis.

The first laser laparoscopy in the UK was performed in October 1982 and we have done over 14,000 operations since then with an excellent safety record and remarkable results. Over a five year study 73 per cent of women reported relief from pain and that their symptoms had lessened after treatment and 80 per cent of women became pregnant.

As with all new developments in surgery these results were met with considerable scepticism from some of our learned academic colleagues and, although they could not contest the fertility data, they suggested that the pain results were based on the patients' desire not to upset us in this new surgical venture. We therefore embarked on the ultimate scientific study – a prospective, randomised, double blind trial in which one group of patients randomly selected by a computer would give informed consent to either having laser treatment or a diagnostic laparoscopy only. They were all followed up with various validated pain scores at six months by a research nurse who was unaware of their treatment. Thus it was double blind since neither the nurse nor the patient was aware of whether the laser had been used. It came as no surprise to me that the results were remarkably similar to our initial five year study and proved beyond a doubt that laser treatment worked in the majority of endometriosis cases and was far more effective than treatment with drugs.

In almost all books and articles about endometriosis the word *enigmatic* appears somewhere in the first paragraph. This essentially means it is puzzling. In spite of a huge amount of research we still do not know the exact cause or whether it is one disease or a medley of several different ones. Some women can be have all the cardinal symptoms with minimal visible disease at laparoscopy, whilst some 5 per cent have severe disease shown when laparoscoped for another reason, such as placing clips on the fallopian tubes to prevent further pregnancies, yet have no pain at all. Other women have classic symptoms of endometriosis yet are found to have irritable bowel syndrome or pelvic venous congestion.

It is therefore not surprising that treatment is confusing and often unsatisfactory and many alternative medical therapies, disciplines and dietary regimes come into play to help the 30 per cent of women where orthodox medicine has failed to relieve the pain or new disease has appeared, often in different places, which is the hallmark of this relentless condition. It is for these sufferers that this book is particularly helpful. All the facts and latest theories are presented in a style that is fluent and easy to read, whilst all the important references to research are cited so the interested reader can follow these up to acquire more detailed knowledge if they so wish.

It is often thought that orthodox doctors disapprove of alternative therapies, but I have always felt that as long as no harm ensues either by creating dangerous side effects, drug interactions or, more importantly, delaying diagnosis of certain treatable cancers, then anything that improves a patient's quality of life and alleviates pain and suffering can only be good. This lively book helps endometriosis sufferers to understand their condition as well as helping them come to terms with it, hopefully leading to symptom relief and an improvement in quality of life to allow them to cope more easily with this strange and ill-understood affliction.

PART 1

THE BACKGROUND

INTRODUCTION

My qualifications for writing about endometriosis are two-fold, as a professional and as a sufferer.

In my work as a nutritional therapist I have met many women suffering from endometriosis, some of whom were previously aware that they had the condition and others who were not. These women might have booked a consultation with me to address seemingly unrelated conditions such as extreme fatigue, depression or painful periods without recognising that these indicated an underlying condition such as endometriosis. Many of these clients had experienced these symptoms for over ten years before being diagnosed.

Their overwhelming feeling is frustration – at often not being heard by the professionals they have seen, at the length of time it took to get diagnosed, at the arguably unnecessary pain they have experienced during this time, and at the lack of information they receive on how to manage the condition once it is diagnosed. I know first-hand just how difficult this can be.

Given that as many as 1 in 10 women are known to suffer from endometriosis, awareness should be significantly greater. On this basis alone I felt inspired to write this book.

I will start with my story.

I did not realise I had endometriosis until I was 26 years old. This came about as a result of studying nutrition. From the start of menstruation at the age of 14 I had suffered severe period pains and bowel discomfort and often felt dizzy and faint.

My first visit to a doctor about these symptoms was at the age of 15. I was prescribed strong painkillers, and the diagnosis was heavy periods (dysmenorrhoea). The painkillers barely made an impact but I was assured that this was the best available treatment.

In the coming years I added chronic tiredness to the list of symptoms and was duly diagnosed with post-viral syndrome. I accepted the heavy periods as something I had to learn to live with, but the extreme fatigue began to interrupt normal teenage living. This continued over the next 14 years with many labels from as many doctors, including chronic fatigue syndrome and myalgic encephalitis (ME).

During my time at university, and indulging in the social scene, I found myself struggling with low mood, increasing lack of energy and pelvic pain, now throughout the month. In retrospect I realise my liver was battling to take on the concoction of a typical student lifestyle and my fluctuating hormones. (More about the connection between the liver and endometriosis later in the book.)

After graduation I sought medical help yet again, explaining that the discomfort was worse and more constant. I was referred for an ultrasound examination. The scan was clear: severe but natural ovulation pain. I felt I had hit a brick wall but remained convinced there was something more to explain my symptoms.

It was not until I began my nutritional training age 25, and was studying the female endocrine (hormonal) system, that I became aware of the hormonal condition endometriosis. On asking my doctor whether this might be my problem, I was told that it was unlikely but if it were, the best options for me were either the contraceptive pill or pregnancy. To quote: 'Is there any real point to investigating it?'

The contraceptive pill was not a route I wanted to go down, and having a child was not an option at that stage in my life. My need for an alternative resolution resulted in my insistence on an investigative procedure known as a laparoscopy. The result showed moderate to severe endometriosis in my left and right fallopian tubes that was likely to have been there since the start of menstruation. After 14 years of going through the mill, I had an answer.

I had laser treatment to remove as much endometrial tissue as was possible. At my post-care check-up I was informed, rather abruptly, that natural fertility was unlikely and I should begin trying to conceive as early as possible. I now understand that

I am one of many thousands of women who are told this potentially devastating news unnecessarily. Having been a strongly maternal person from an early age I felt deeply upset by this prospect. I was determined to take my health into my own hands, to improve my everyday well-being and to challenge the prognosis of possible infertility.

I used diet and realistic lifestyle changes that I knew I could stick to. These did not involve living in a cave, yoga for an hour each day or avoiding any form of normal life. Instead I just became more conscious of my health in general: eating delicious foods and drinking lovely wine but in moderation. A year later things were very different, my endometriosis felt a lot calmer and, having married, I began trying for a baby. Four months later I discovered I was pregnant with our first son Alfie, born in 2007, and in 2010, after another natural conception and healthy pregnancy, I had our second son Ned.

Nowadays my endometriosis is manageable, with months going by where my pain is minimal, if present at all. I have had no fainting, no bowel discomfort, my energy has improved remarkably and I continue to eat responsibly and take care of myself. I know there are particular dietary triggers that if I choose to eat or drink can affect my well-being. Sometimes I still opt to indulge in these and other times I don't. This is my choice but it is an informed one. Eating and living truly well is not a chore, it is a genuine pleasure. I say this is not because I am a nutritionist; I say this because I am a woman who has now experienced the physical and emotional rewards of valuing and respecting the body's amazing ability to heal when given the right tools.

In this book I share with you the experience and knowledge of this condition, not only my own, but also that of the inspiring individuals I have had the pleasure to work with and learn from along the way. Most importantly, I cannot make you well; that bit is down to you. But I will guide and nurture you through the approach stage by stage. I urge you to dedicate the time and effort to embrace it fully and value your body; it can be the smallest changes that make a significant difference to how you feel. By taking control, you can work with your body to achieve the wellness and improvement that I already know. Feeling powerless is crushingly disheartening and can leave you feeling depressed and low; it does not need to be this way.

I have had the enlightening privilege to work alongside Professor Chris Sutton in writing this book and his pearls of wisdom have contributed a great deal throughout, but most especially in Chapter 1. This chapter looks at the physiology of endometriosis and current medical approaches. In my experience women are often diagnosed with the condition and leave the consultant's room with little or no clarification about what endometriosis is. They may not have had an explanation as to which line of treatment is best suited to them, or, if they have been recommended a course of treatment, they may leave without knowledge of either the side effects or the benefits of such treatment. I hope that this chapter can offer you some clarity. In Chapter 2 I explain the powerful role that food and lifestyle can play in the management of endometriosis. We will look a little more into the areas of the body that need to be supported in this disease and why this is. Chapters 3 and 4 look at the approach of living and eating consciously to support the body and healing process. Chapter 5 is a practical chapter giving tips on how to put theory into practice. My aim is not to bombard you with 'what not to do's' but to offer a positive, practical and nurturing way of eating and living that can easily fit into the parameters of your everyday life.

Chapters 6 and 7 look at the benefits of 'kickstarting' the body's own discovery of balanced health and how to do this. Chapter 8 looks at other areas of health that will benefit from following this approach, and the protective role this has on your future. The useful contacts offered in Part 5 have all been selected personally and I can highly recommend all of them.

The key to making these changes is to invest in the process fully. I would love to guarantee that every woman who follows this approach will be fully healed from endometriosis, but sadly neither I nor anyone else can give this promise. However, what I can offer are the tools of awareness and knowledge. I hope that you use these to empower you, so that you, like many of the women I have worked with, can experience vast improvements in your endometriosis now and in the years to come.

MY APPROACH TO NUTRITIONAL THERAPY

I remain amazed by the natural power of food. Any lasting and healing approach to disease has to look at what goes in, what goes out and all the bits in between! The body has to be viewed as a whole rather than simply by addressing the superficial symptoms. Effective nutritional therapy looks at the root causes in order to rediscover natural balance.

My driving force is a desire to understand the human being as a whole, the soul, the emotions, the environment, the functions of the body and their integrative role to maximise health. It is easy to think of yourself as a victim, misunderstood and ignored by health professionals in whom you have placed your trust. I hope that this book shares with you the information to change this way of thinking, to re-charge you with the power, knowledge and motivation to take control. Use your experience as an opportunity to flourish, rather than holding you back from living life to the full.

Henrietta Norton, Dip Raw NT, MBANT, BSc

WHAT IS ENDOMETRIOSIS? 1

Despite being one of the most common gynaecological diseases, the cause of endometriosis remains controversial. It is estimated that approximately 10–15 per cent of all premenopausal women have endometriosis. Sixty per cent of these women are diagnosed when aged 25–35 years old but 43 per cent of this group experienced the start of symptoms in their teenage years. Some cases produce overt symptoms whilst others show none.[1]

Endometriosis can continue undiagnosed indefinitely in some individuals, their cyclical discomfort accepted as part of the standard course of menstruation. Even women who have known about their endometriosis for years may still be unsure what endometriosis is exactly. This is understandable; medical professionals find it confusing too.

Endometriosis is a complex disorder of the female reproductive tract. It affects women of childbearing age regardless of race. The derivation of the name is *endo* (inside) and *metra* (uterus). Endometrial cells that usually live inside the uterus (hereafter referred to as the womb), and which form the lining, sneak outside this usual habitat and migrate to other areas of the body. They choose the parts they like the most and, like ex-pats, settle there making their new home and compound. The most common 'destinations' are the lower part of the pelvis – the ovaries, fallopian tubes, bladder, rectum, surface of the womb and the 'cul-de-sac' (the space behind the womb, also called the pouch of Douglas). More rarely they will travel to the upper parts of the abdomen (sitting above the pelvis), including the small intestine, stomach, kidney and diaphragm. Typically, endometriosis occurs on the pelvic structures, but may occur in virtually any part of the body and in multiple locations. The most random place of endometriosis growth I have had experience of in clinic is the nostrils.

Once settled, they become patches (medically, these are called implants or lesions, but I think patches illustrates them better). Under a microscope, they look very similar to the lining of the womb. So similar are they, that they are hormonally connected to the lining of the womb. This means they experience the same fluctuations in hormones and therefore also shed or bleed at the time of menstruation. As this blood loss often occurs in a confined space, or compound to continue the analogy, without the outlet of the cervix or vagina, it can cause swelling and extreme pain. If this occurs in the ileosacral joints (the muscles, tissue and bone in the pelvis) it can also cause discomfort in the leg and back muscles. This is why most women find the pain is either only at the time of menstruation or is worse at that time.

As the word 'patches' suggests, they are sticky and so hang on for dear life when they find their chosen resting place.

The body is well equipped to heal itself and you might therefore think that it would be efficient at correcting this situation. But this natural healing process can, conversely, make the problem worse. The body forms protective scar tissue around the patches, just as it does for a scrape on the skin. Think of a scar on your skin that you may have and then you can picture how it would feel on the inside of your body.

The organs within the pelvis and abdomen live within close proximity. A combination of this plus the naturally bumpy surface of the scar and the sticky consistency of the patches themselves can cause some of the organs to stick together – rather like a cobweb. These patches are known as 'adhesions' in the medical world. Adhesions can create a tugging effect, feeling tight on those organs, and can cause pain. Women with endometriosis often describe a 'tugging' or 'dragging' effect and this is perhaps why.

These irritating patches grow and spread in the presence of a key female hormone: oestrogen. Would the obvious solution be to cut off the supply of this hormone? Well even if this was possible, these devious patches are also thought to produce their own 'home-brew' of oestrogen, perpetuating the cycle further.[2] Fat cells also produce oestrogen, so keeping your body fat percentage within the healthy range is important. This can be measured using an indicator called the Body Mass Index (BMI). This tries to identify the percentage of body tissue that is actually fat. There are disadvantages to this method, as it does not take into consideration our individual variation of bone, muscle, fat and organs but it provides a broader range for what is considered to be normal. A BMI score of 18.5–24.9 is seen as the 'healthy range'. One of the best and most convenient ways to measure body fat is to use an electronic machine that uses bioelectrical impedance. It may sound confusing but it is actually quite a simple method. An electrical current (don't worry you won't feel it!) is passed through the body and the machine measures how long it takes for the current to come out. Lean tissue is a much better conductor of electricity than fatty tissue and therefore the machine is able to measure the percentage of body fat. All of these points are discussed in more detail throughout the book.

As well as producing oestrogen, these patches have the capacity to secrete other chemical substances called prostaglandins. Prostaglandins are a group of natural chemicals regulating our experience of pain and are released by the lining of the womb as well as elsewhere in the body. Usually the lining of the womb secretes these chemicals, which are then expelled through the vagina, whereas, when distributed by the patches of endometriosis, they have no escape route. With little option the body then has to dump these chemicals anywhere it can and this may result in adverse effects. These can include swelling, increased or decreased gut motility (irritable bowel syndrome) and interruption of a healthy reproductive cycle.

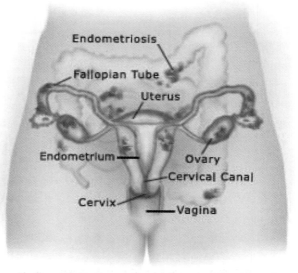

Endometriosis

Endometriosis

Fallopian Tube

Uterus

Endometrium

Ovary

Cervical Canal

Cervix

Vagina

Endometriosis occurs when endometrial cells, normally found only on the inside of the uterus travels backwards through the fallopian tubes and become embedded in locations outside the uterus.

The American Society for Reproductive Medicine has defined four stages of endometriosis that you may see on your patient notes if you have been diagnosed with endometriosis (see page 10 for an illustration).[3]

STAGE 1–Endometriosis in stage 1 is classified as minimal, meaning that there are isolated patches of endometrial tissue growth outside the womb. Stages 1 and 2 are peritoneal. The peritoneum is a layer made up of cells, blood vessels and a lymphatic capillary network that covers the abdominal and pelvic walls and organs.

STAGE 2–Endometriosis in stage 2 is considered mild. A doctor makes this diagnosis when there are several small patches and a few small areas of scar tissue or adhesions.

STAGE 3–Stage 3 is moderate. The patches are both superficial and deep. There are also several prominent areas of scar tissue or adhesions. Typically the physical symptoms of endometriosis are present in patients with moderate stage 3 endometriosis. Stages 3 and 4 usually have chocolate cysts – cysts with old blood inside hence the dark brown appearance (or endometriomas).

STAGE 4–This is the most severe stage of endometriosis. Patients with stage 4 will have many superficial and deep implants as well as large adhesions. Intense pelvic pain and reduced fertility are common. This stage usually has deep infiltrating endometriosis that most often involves deep pelvic structures such as uterosacral ligaments (the supporting ligament connecting the sacrum and the cervix), cul-de-sac (the space just above the vagina between the rectosigmoid colon and cervix), apex of the vagina, the tissue between the rectum and vagina, rectosigmoid colon, pelvic sidewalls, ovaries, fallopian tubes and bladder. When the infiltration of endometriosis becomes this deep, the patches are regulated by bloodstream factors making it harder to control their growth.

WHAT DOES ENDOMETRIOSIS LOOK LIKE?

Like human beings, patches of endometriosis come in a variety of shapes, sizes and colours. These different colours may reflect different stages of the condition. Young women in the early stages of endometriosis (before it has developed scar tissue) are more likely to have clear, pink or red lesions. Unfortunately because of their clever camouflage they are also the trickier patches to recognise during medical investigations such as laparoscopy (more on this later). Older women with the condition are likely to have had the condition for a while and therefore their patches of endometriosis tend to be a brownish black colour, or in the latter stages, white (you will see why below). Some women can have a patchwork combination (see illustration page 13).[4]

So appearance of the patches is varied and below is a list of the different ways they can appear:

RED PATCHES

These patches are red in colour because they are filled with little blood vessels. Just like the toddler equivalent in humans, these young patches are the most active and may well be the main cause of pain and 'swelling' around the affected area. They also have a very active oestrogen home-brew department. These tend to be in the first stages of endometriosis. They are like blisters (albeit blisters are in fact white). I am sure you can now picture why they cause the discomfort: just as blisters on a foot irritate and cause pain so too do these. These patches are most common in younger women.

CLEAR PATCHES

These too look like little blisters and are common in the early stages of endometriosis. They do not contain any blood vessels, hence their opaque appearance. As you can imagine, these are hard to detect during internal investigations and therefore may be part of the reason why so many women remain undiagnosed by procedures such as ultrasound.

BLACK PATCHES

By the time patches appear black they are rendered inactive, their factory of home-brew hormones and chemicals virtually closed down. This is at the stage when scar tissue has occurred and the scarring has blocked the blood vessels, trapping the blood and giving it a black appearance. These patches are also known as powder burn patches and are most common in older women.

WHITE PATCHES

Over time, the body absorbs the black matter within the patches and leaves a thick white scar. The white tissue indicates the presence of deep infiltrating disease and the deeper it infiltrates the more painful it is either by invading sensory nerves, especially in the utero-sacral ligaments (the major ligaments of the uterus) or by the fibro-muscular hyperplasia.

Most patches are thin and small at about 1–2mm in diameter but when endometriosis has progressed to the third or fourth stage, women can also develop another larger 'morph' of endometriosis, chocolate cysts.

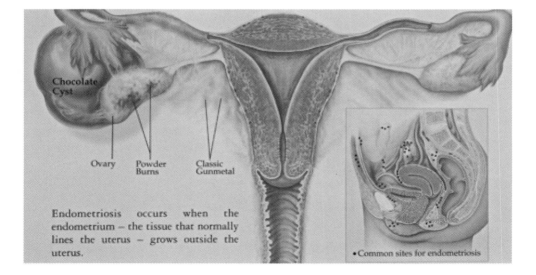

Chocolate Cyst

Ovary   Powder   Classic
         Burns   Gunmetal

Endometriosis occurs when the endometrium – the tissue that normally lines the uterus – grows outside the uterus.

• Common sites for endometriosis

CHOCOLATE CYSTS

A cyst simply means a space with fluid in it. Sadly chocolate cysts are not filled with chocolate as the name would suggest (this might make the condition a lot more palatable!) but with old blood. These are larger lumps of endometriosis that grow inside an ovary. They may be several centimetres across and the fluid content is dark brown colour. Chocolate cysts occur at the later development stage of endometriosis,

WHAT IS A HORMONE?–'Hormone' derives from the Greek word meaning to 'urge on'. Aptly named, hormones are carried in the blood to trigger activities in the body. The reproductive hormones, including oestrogen and progesterone, control women's monthly menstrual cycle and pregnancy.

WHAT IS OESTROGEN?–This is an umbrella term for a group of hormones. Most health experts use the term 'oestrogen' as a term to cover all oestrogens. For the sake of simplicity, we only use the term oestrogen.

WHAT IS OVULATION?–This is the stage of a woman's reproductive cycle in which an egg is released by a part of the ovary known as a follicle, which then travels down the fallopian tubes. This usually occurs 14 days before the end of the cycle (the start of menstruation).

WHAT IS PROGESTERONE?–This is a hormone manufactured in the ovaries and adrenal glands that promotes the growth of the lining of the womb during the last half of the menstrual cycle to prepare for pregnancy, referred to as the 'luteal phase'. It plays a major role in regulating the menstrual cycle. It enhances mood, helps protect against certain cancers, and reduces or stops bone loss (osteoporosis).

WHAT IS THE PITUITARY GLAND?–Located at the base of the brain just below the hypothalamus, this gland controls many major hormonal factories throughout the body including the testicles, ovaries, adrenal glands and the thyroid gland.

meaning that if these are present then endometriosis has been around in the body for a few years. The technical term for these cysts is endometrioma.

WHAT ARE THE CAUSES OF ENDOMETRIOSIS?

Endometriosis can affect all women of childbearing age. The typical woman with endometriosis has been described as in her thirties, a career minded woman who has delayed childbearing. While we know this is far from the truth, the myth persists. Rather, it is most likely that a woman does not discover she has endometriosis until fertility is a concern, and that this is nowadays in the early to mid-thirties on average.

I wish I could say otherwise but it is unknown what exactly causes this mysterious condition. As so many women suffer from it this may sound as unbelievable to you as it does to me, but research continues and several possibilities have been suggested:

GENETICS

It has been proposed that the beginning of endometriosis occurs during foetal development when young endometrial cells are displaced. These then begin to grow on reaching puberty. Evidence suggests that neither oestrogen nor progesterone are required for the implantation and early growth of the endometrial cells, although on reaching puberty, when these hormones are stimulated, progression can occur.[5] It appears that those women with a first-degree relative (mother or sister) with endometriosis are up to nine times more likely to experience this themselves and are equally more likely to have it severely.[6,7] This would explain why endometriosis tends to run in families.

OESTROGEN DOMINANCE

This is certainly an extremely popular theory for the progression of endometriosis, if not a co-factor in its initiation too. Many women with endometriosis have a dominance of oestrogen where the level of this hormone is out of balance with the level of progesterone. The balance between these two hormones is essential for optimum hormonal and reproductive health. A dominance of oestrogen may be a result of environmental toxins, a weakened detoxification system and a reduced ability of the body to bring back hormonal equilibrium. This dominance is thought to encourage the growth and development of endometriosis until oestrogen levels are balanced by management strategies. This theory also supports the metaplasia theory outlined next.

METAPLASIA THEORY

This simply means cells changing from a normal cell structure into an abnormal cell structure according to their environment, a little like a chameleon. This theory suggests that cells in the body can change structure and function to become endometrial cells when influenced by a particular environment.[8] For example, metaplasia can be triggered if there is a surge of oestrogen during puberty or by being exposed to environmental xeno-oestrogens. Xeno-oestrogens are found in a vast array of our foods nowadays and in the production and packaging of many foods. They have a similar structure to natural oestrogens and the body recognises them as such. This means that when they are present the body reacts to them as oestrogens. As a result there may be an increase in circulating oestrogen, disrupting the crucial balance with progesterone further still. This theory was underpinned by an interesting study that found endometrial patches in the bladders of men being treated for prostate cancer with oestrogenic drugs.[9] I'll discuss this in more detail in Part 2.

WHAT ARE XENO-OESTROGENS?–Xeno-oestrogens are synthetic industrial chemicals found in pesticides, fuels, drugs and polycarbonate plastic bottles and food containers. They cause hormonal activity similar to oestrogen and may alter the natural form of the hormone made by the body. Avoiding xeno-oestrogens has a positive impact on female health and these will be discussed more in Chapter 2.

THE INFLUENCE OF MENSTRUATION ITSELF

Women with short monthly cycles (less than 27 days) and long bleeding time (more than 7 days) have twice the risk of developing endometriosis.[10]

Young women and girls are experiencing the onset of menstruation at an increasingly early age. This exposes the female population to more years of menstruation, with use of bleached tampons and environmental synthetic hormones from the contraceptive pill for example. Could this see a worrying increase in the incidence of endometriosis? Although this is theory at the moment I believe it to be a cause for concern and one that requires greater investigation.

DELAYED CHILDBEARING

Although the term 'delayed childbearing' is a controversial one these days, feminist opinions aside, it can have a significant influence on the progression of endometriosis. Hormones produced during pregnancy and breastfeeding have a protective effect on the womb and temporarily stop menstruation. This in turn reduces the frequency of periods in a woman's life. If childbearing is delayed (categorised as late thirties and older), and the onset of menstruation is getting younger, the frequency of menstruation becomes greater.[11] But this suggests that delayed childbearing is a choice. In some cases pregnancy has not been possible or endometriosis is not discovered until a woman attempts to become pregnant and, because the endometriosis has had a longer period in which to progress, fertility may have become impaired. This is a tricky issue and one I will touch on in more detail later in the book.

RETROGRADE THEORY

The most clinically supported theory is retrograde menstruation, a concept proposed by Dr Sampson more than 90 years ago.[12] Although endometriotic cysts had been described before by W.W. Russell in 1898, Dr Sampson, a gynaecologist, studied the disease systematically and in 1921 proposed that endometriosis – a term he coined – was a result of 'retrograde menstruation'. Also known as 'transplantation theory', it proposes that endometriosis is due to endometrial tissue abnormally flowing up the fallopian tubes in the blood and into the abdomen or bowel. Retrograde menstruation appears to occur in almost all women to one degree or another, but in women with endometriosis it seems to be worse. Obstruction of the flow and exit of blood from the cervix has been blamed for this, as has poor muscle tone around the junction of the fallopian tubes and the womb.[13] The use of tampons has been linked to this theory as they can interfere with the free flow of the blood from the body.

LYMPH TRANSPORT

It is also known that parts of the endometrial tissue can be carried to other parts of the body by the lymph or blood circulatory system. This does not account for why the endometrial tissue exists in the first place but does explain how it appears in very random places on occasion, such as the fingernails – I kid you not.[14]

WEAKENED IMMUNE FUNCTION

A weakened immune system also appears to have a significant impact. What is not known is whether this is a symptom or a cause of endometriosis. The immune system sees endometriosis as a threat and reacts by stimulating inflammation in that area as a means of protection. As endometriosis is ever-present, this means the immune system thinks it is continually 'under attack' and can become overworked and weakened. It is also proposed that the immune system in a woman with endometriosis is less able to clear the 'debris' from menstruation as effectively as those without, therefore 'fuelling' the endometriosis patches further.[15] Weakened immune defences can also occur as a result of chronic stress, poor diet, nutritional deficiencies and poor digestive health. This is discussed in more detail in Part 2.

In all theories, endometriosis is regarded as a progressive disease, graduating from minimal to severe stages if left unmanaged. It would seem that genetic inheritance, and delaying childbearing, which increases the exposure to menstruation, appear to enhance the development of the disease but this does not explain its presence in the first place.[16] As so often with hormonal conditions, I feel endometriosis is a melting pot of all the factors discussed and each one needs to be addressed for any treatment to be effective. For example, a genetic predisposition may not be enough for endometriosis to develop *unless* exposed to environmental risk factors such as the xeno-oestrogen dioxin.[17] Throughout the book I will look at how these factors can be dealt with naturally and practically.

WHAT ARE THE SYMPTOMS?

What is so fascinating and frustrating about endometriosis is that the severity of the symptoms is not always relative to the degree of the disease. Some with advanced endometriosis suffer no discomfort, whereas others with a mild degree of the condition can be in extreme pain. There may be no symptoms at all or a combination of several such as varied or heavy bleeding, bowel and bladder symptoms, depression and fatigue. The experience of the symptoms is really only a reflection of where in the body endometriosis has decided to harbour itself.

You may understand a little more now why there is such difficulty in diagnosis and in estimating accurately the amount of women suffering from endometriosis.

PAIN

Pain during a period or pain throughout the cycle is reported by 95 per cent of women with endometriosis.[18] Pain is a natural response to jolt the body into a healing, reactive state when something is wrong. Triggering this healing response causes the immune system to release its army of natural chemicals to the area in strife, including prostaglandin 1 (PGE1). Once there, they build a protective layer around the problem area by inflaming it – swelling rather like an air bag in a car. It also causes the muscles in the area to tighten. All of this can put weight and pressure on nerve endings, stimulating more pain.

Other pain may be caused by adhesions (organs sticking together), as mentioned earlier. Clients of mine have also described this as a 'dragging feeling'. The pain associated with endometriosis is in an altogether different league from 'normal' period pain. It can be debilitating and disrupt your everyday tasks, including work. Suffered regularly it can be exhausting both mentally and physically.

When the body is relaxed it is able to counter this pain cycle by releasing clever chemicals from the brain that are natural painkillers; these are called endorphins. However, experiencing pain to any degree can be unsettling and this makes us feel tense, setting up physical stress.

In Part 2 we look at the powerful contributory role that food choices can play in both increasing and significantly reducing experience of inflammation and therefore associated pain.

Pain is subjective but here are some examples of where and how pain may occur.

Severe pelvic pain and cramping

This pain can be independent of, or accompanied by, a period or ovulation when the egg is passing down from the ovary into the fallopian tube (usually 14 days before a period). Pain due to endometriosis during ovulation or between periods is commonly felt in the same spot. Women have described the pain as a 'dragging sensation' or a 'knotted feeling'.

Pain with intercourse

The medical term for this is 'dyspareunia'. It is a keynote symptom that alerts doctors to a possible diagnosis of endometriosis. This symptom is reported to feature in up to 64 per cent of all women with endometriosis.[19] Aside from the physical pain it can also be emotionally challenging with the associated frustration and guilt that can arise from not being able to enjoy sex. This is especially true in modern society where the media can encourage women to feel like failures if they are not sexual goddesses. The pain can be felt deep inside and may be worse in certain sexual positions. Ironically natural chemicals released in the body during pleasurable pastimes such as sex can also reduce pain – it's just getting to the pleasure stage that is the problem.

Painful periods

The medical term for this is 'dysmenorrhoea'. It is associated with the confined internal bleeding characteristic of endometriosis. Pain usually lasts beyond the first couple of days of the period and may even begin leading up to the period. Typically a woman suffering from endometriosis will also experience lower back pain in these days. This is probably because moderate and severe endometriosis adhesions have developed among organs and this puts extra pressure on bones and muscles around the lower back.

BLEEDING

Spotting between periods

This can occur at any point during the cycle and may be red fresh blood or a darker brown colour. Many of my clients have told me they experience spotting three or four days after their period has finished or before their period begins. This is due to the fluctuating level of hormones. The endometrial patches produce so many hormones and chemicals that it is no surprise this happens.

Heavy bleeding
Heavy bleeding during a regular period is common and can include blood clots. Heavy bleeding outside a period is unusual and it is important a doctor rules out any other cause.

Irregular periods
Prolonged bleeding, longer than five days, or irregular cycles of menstruation is a result of the abnormal fluctuation of hormones.

Loss of large blood clots during menstruation
Natural chemicals that can cause the blood to clot and increase flow are released as a protective response to the pain and inflammation.

Bleeding from the bowel
Although patches of endometriosis are common in the bowel it is important not to assume that the bleeding is due to endometriosis until other conditions have been excluded. Check with your doctor.

BLADDER AND BOWEL SYMPTOMS
Discomfort in the bowel
Patches of endometriosis are common in the bowel in moderate to severe endometriosis. Abdominal discomfort is reported by 84 per cent of women with endometriosis, causing pain and interrupting the healthy functions of the bowel.[20] Prostaglandins produced as a response to the immune system also affect the digestive system and can result in cramping, pain on passing stools, constipation, bloating, diarrhoea or nausea. As the gut is so closely linked to the mind, mental tension as a result of the endometriosis can also put pressure on the health of the bowel. The gut is sometimes referred to as the second brain (it has the same nerve receptors as the brain hence butterflies in your stomach when nervous), so it is no

wonder that the stress of endometriosis also affects digestive health. See Part 2 for more detail on the gut link.

Bladder discomfort
This can occur when patches of endometriosis have attached themselves to the bladder wall or when adhesions are present and sticking the bladder to other organs. This can make the simple task of urinating uncomfortable. Again, it is very important to check with your doctor, as this can also be a symptom of other conditions such as a urinary tract infection.

OTHER SYMPTOMS
Reduced immune defences
The immune system in sufferers of endometriosis is impaired.[21] Whether or not this is a symptom or a cause is debatable.

SUB-FERTILITY OR INFERTILITY
This subject deserves a book in its own right but is described in more detail in Part 2 where I distinguish sub-fertility from infertility. While endometriosis is common in women who experience infertility, infertility is certainly not an experience of every sufferer of endometriosis. Far from it: many women with endometriosis become pregnant easily. Some studies have shown that it might take longer to achieve pregnancy in women with endometriosis than those without the disease but it is well known that intervention is often not needed.[22] Endometriosis can all too often be blamed for infertility when in fact there other factors at play too. In one comprehensive study an impressive 80 per cent of women became pregnant after treatment with laparoscopy when no other infertility factors were involved.[23] Women with chocolate cysts may be *sub*-fertile (where fertility is impaired or sub optimum rather than irreparable or permanent) because the cysts distort the shape of the fallopian tubes making it difficult for the finger-like ends to pick up an egg. However, once the cyst is removed and the tube returned to its normal size, and dye used to check its flow, a good pregnancy rate can follow (one study states that 57 per cent of patients became pregnant within 6–9 months of the procedure).[24]

Environmental xeno-oestrogens (see page 43), in food and the environment, have been shown to disrupt the production of and use of natural progesterone manufactured by the body. The way in which these chemicals interrupt this process also disrupts the balanced environment of the womb necessary to achieve pregnancy.[25] Research indicates that this may be an influential factor in the occurrence of miscarriage or reduced ability to conceive.[26]

DEPRESSION/LOW MOODS

Sufferers of endometriosis report increased occurrence of symptoms of premenstrual syndrome such as depression, low mood, sore breasts and irritability. This may be caused by the abnormal levels of oestrogen but may also be influenced by the anxiety and distress this condition can bring. Oestrogen levels are linked with the 'feel good hormone' serotonin that can therefore be reduced resulting in a susceptibility to mild depression. Equally, depression understandably occurs with most diseases of chronic pain. It seems to evolve as the disease and discomfort progress and can be part of the overall distress of the patient.[27] Add to this the journey it may have taken to reach diagnosis and depression can become more likely.

TIREDNESS

Tiredness is, of course, subjective and this makes it hard to identify what is 'appropriate' tiredness from daily life and what is over and above this. A surprising 87 per cent of women with endometriosis reported exhaustion and low energy; this high statistic indicates this is much more than just a coincidence.[28]

Ranging from extreme, inexplicable fatigue to a general lethargy that can be constant or intermittent, there is no easy explanation why women with endometriosis often feel so tired. It may be that when the body is in a state of disease and the immune system 'activated' all energy is focused on the area in need of healing. If this is a continual state (as it is in the case of endometriosis) energy supply to the rest of the body is less. Pain itself is very wearing, as is the stress and worry involved in trying to continue with a normal life despite everything mentioned above.

WHAT IS NITRIC OXIDE?–A natural and necessary body chemical, which can become excessive if the immune system is weakened.

MIGRAINE

Recent research shows that women with endometriosis may be as much as doubly susceptible to experiencing migraine.[29] The frequency or degree of migraine is not related to how severe the endometriosis is but researchers have found migraines start earlier in life in young women who have endometriosis than those who do not – 16.4 years as opposed to 21.9.[30] The link between the two conditions is not really understood although some biochemical mediators have been implicated. It is possible that prostaglandin 1 (PGE1) produced and spread by endometriosis may contribute to migraine and it has also been shown that high nitric oxide synthesis has a role in both migraines and endometriosis. But the association between the two conditions requires further research.

Symptoms, particularly pain, are not just a direct result of endometriosis. Rather they are a combination of the very presence of endometriosis and the knock-on effect of the condition. I feel that the condition cannot only be managed but also improved by combining surgery to remove the endometriosis and natural management techniques to heal the damage, re-establish hormonal balance and truly support the immune and reproductive system.

HOW IS ENDOMETRIOSIS DIAGNOSED AND TREATED?

Getting a sympathetic diagnosis of endometriosis is too often the biggest obstacle of this condition. This is partly because there is no reliable blood test that can be used and even the most commonly recommended ultrasound methods can be misleading. The only foolproof way to diagnose the condition is having a laparoscopy as this precise procedure leaves no room for a missed diagnosis and in my experience most women who undergo a laparoscopy discover they have endometriosis. I have also found from personal and professional experience that assertiveness is the name of game when asking for this procedure: a patient can request any investigatory process that she feels she needs. My number one piece of advice is to trust your instinct and if you feel something isn't right, push for the answers. Do not be fobbed off.

LAPAROSCOPY
Laparoscopy is a surgical procedure that involves placing a laparoscope through an incision in the navel with one to three 5mm incisions just above the pubic bone. This is the only method currently available to diagnose endometriosis accurately, and determine where it is present, its nature (e.g. chocolate cysts) and the degree of it. Typically if endometriosis is found following a investigative laparoscopy, treatment will require a further laparoscopy to perform endometrial ablation to remove as much of it as possible. To avoid this double procedure, you may ask your surgeon beforehand to remove anything found there and then rather than having to undergo further surgery. (Sometimes this is not possible.)

I fully support the surgical removal of the endometrial patches as a first-line defence in halting or removing the disease. It sets the stage for natural methods to get to work in achieving and maintaining hormonal equilibrium. Evidence shows that women who have the operation feel the optimum benefit after six months. Interestingly, the first three months can feel as though the operation has made no difference; perhaps this is because the body has to repair the trauma associated with any surgery.[31] Studies have shown that 70 per cent of patients who had suffered from pain previously were pain-free after the operation and in one study 45 of the 56 patients (80 per cent) presenting with infertility due to endometriosis alone became pregnant.[32,33]

Laparoscopy involves using a laser or diathermy (intense heat) to remove or burn off the patches of endometriosis. The procedure is performed under general anaesthetic and only requires a small incision through the navel and possibly one either side near the hip bones to check the ovaries and fallopian tubes. Gas (carbon dioxide) is used to inflate the area to get a better view. Post-operatively a small amount of gas may still be left inside and cause discomfort as it tries to make its way out of the body. A common complaint is shoulder ache, a reflective pain from gas being trapped under the diaphragm.

The laser or diathermy technique can work well for chocolate cysts, where the surgeon will pierce the chocolate cyst to remove the liquid matter (old blood) inside it. Adhesions can also be removed but there is the risk of further scar tissue. To prevent this from happening some surgeons use protective membranes to separate the organs, leaving them in place.

A laparoscopy can also detect endometrial lesions in other areas of the abdominal cavity, such as on the outside of the lower bowel and appendix. Adequate surgical excision of the deep infiltrating endometriosis provides the best long-term results and symptomatic relief. Because of the deep invasive nature of the disease and the frequency of the disease involving the vital pelvic organs, the gynaecologist must be experienced and competent in performing bowel, bladder and ureteral surgery.

A much newer procedure similar to the laser laparoscopy is the PlasmaJet using Argon Neutral Plasma Energy, a by-product of Russian space technology with tissue effects almost identical to the carbon dioxide laser. For more information on this see Plasma surgical in the Useful Contacts section (page 166).

HELICA THERMAL COAGULATOR
This is a procedure that involves a helium beam that heats the surface of the

LOOK AFTER YOURSELF AFTER SURGERY: If surgery is your chosen option to begin management of your endometriosis, make sure you get plenty of rest after the surgery. Usually you can be in and out of hospital within the same day but it can take up to a week to recover fully. It is vital that you allow your body the period of rest it deserves after an operation. Drink plenty of fluids, sleep as much as your body needs and eat a diet rich in vegetables and fruit to boost the nutrients needed for optimum recovery. Take a high-strength multi-nutrient that contains antioxidants (see Chapter 4) to speed the healing process and bring you maximum post-operative benefits. Vitamin E and rosehip oil creams and oils are excellent at reducing scarring. Start the Kickstart and Nurture diets about a month after the operation.

endometrial tissues, causing them to dry out. The dry tissue is then reabsorbed into the system without forming a scab. This process has been criticised as researchers have failed to publish trials and clinical efficacy data to prove how effective it really is.

ULTRASOUND

Most endometriosis cannot be picked up by an ultrasound scan. This is because the endometriosis is too 'thin' to be seen as a change to the pelvic surface by the ultrasound. The exception to the rule is a chocolate cyst which looks grainy, giving it a unique appearance on the scan.

YOU KNOW YOUR BODY BEST

If you are the one with the pain and/or concerns then regardless of what your family, friends or doctor might say, if your symptoms are a problem for you and other treatments have not worked then you should look further. You may not have endometriosis but trust your judgement and respect your right to know what is going on in your body.

It is not appropriate to perform a laparoscopy on every girl or woman who complains to her doctor about pain in the pelvic region. But it is essential to determine a diagnosis. The choice is always down to you and you need to weigh up the benefits of having the investigation done compared with the degree of the symptoms that you are feeling.

HYSTERECTOMY

This is perhaps the most extreme treatment offered for endometriosis and is thankfully less commonly used than it was (although arguably still too commonly). In the case of endometriosis it is usually both the womb and the ovaries that are removed. Once the ovaries are removed the woman will go into the menopause literally overnight. In contrast to the natural menopause where the hormone levels decline gently over time, a surgically induced menopause by hysterectomy is a huge shock to the body. The

A NOTE ON OMEGA 3 ESSENTIAL FATTY ACIDS: If you are planning on having an operation, research[34] has shown that the omega 3 fatty acid EPA, taken five days before the scheduled operation, can have a positive impact on inflammation after the operation, reducing infection, improving wound healing and shortening recovery time.[35]

sudden loss of oestrogen can be a risk factor in developing osteoporosis. Following a hysterectomy the woman may be offered hormone replacement therapy (HRT) patches to reduce the symptoms. If this is an oestrogel or oestrogen skin patch replaced at six month intervals, or an oestrogen/testosterone implant the disease will not reactivate. However, combined HRT with progesterone will fuel any patches of endometriosis that are located elsewhere in the body such as the bowel.

STEM CELL RESEARCH

Stem cell isolation and its potential role in the treatment of endometriosis is a hot, and to date, incomplete area of gynaecological research.[36] The lining of the womb undergoes cycles of growth and regression with each menstrual cycle. Certain stem cells that reside in the womb (progenitor stem cells) are thought to be responsible for this regenerative capacity, but they may also have the ability to generate endometriosis. Another type of stem cell (mesenchymal stem cell) is also believed to be involved in the development of endometriosis. Recent publications have identified multipotent stem cells in the endometrium that are useful in tissue engineering and regenerative medicine.[37] It is thought that by isolating these different types the development and treatment of endometriosis can be very specific and managed extremely effectively. It is an area that needs and is receiving a lot of research and attention; I would be surprised if this does not become a first-line approach to treating endometriosis in the next ten years.

PRESCRIPTION MEDICATION FOR ENDOMETRIOSIS
THE CONTRACEPTIVE PILL

This pill is a combination of oestrogen and progesterone. It tricks the body into thinking it is pregnant. The monthly bleed is not a genuine period but a reaction to a drop in synthetic hormones within the pill. This method has been shown to arrest the symptoms or progression of endometriosis but only superficially; the condition remains present in the body. If the contraceptive pill is stopped the symptoms return. The contraceptive pill can cause side effects such as headaches, bloating and nutritional deficiencies. Sometimes the pill is used at high doses to stop bleeding completely but this can cause even harsher side effects such as vomiting, blood clots, low sex drive and depression.

PROGESTERONE-ONLY PILL

This pill uses a synthetic version of the hormone progesterone only and can also trick the body into thinking it is pregnant. The side effects of this can include nausea, weight gain, tender breasts and low energy.

DANAZOL

Like all the other hormonal treatments, danazol does not cure endometriosis permanently. Rather it suppresses its growth and development temporarily, so the disease may recur following treatment. This is the main drug prescribed for endometriosis and it uses a synthetically modified version of testosterone. This prevents ovulation and in turn prevents the lining of the womb developing or thickening, suppressing the growth of endometrial implants and causing them to degenerate. Danazol is usually taken orally but a vaginal ring containing the drug, which can limit side effects, is also available. Side effects are common and can be extreme; in some women they can include mood swings, dizziness, headaches, increased sex drive, facial hair, acne and weight gain to name a few.

GONADOTROPHIN RELEASING HORMONE ANALOGUES (GnRH)

These are synthetic hormones that can be sprayed up the nose, implanted under the skin or injected. They put the body into a temporary menopause by stopping the ovaries from producing certain hormones that in turn reduce levels of oestrogen in the blood. This decline in oestrogen has been shown to shrink endometriosis patches. But it comes at a steep price by stimulating the symptoms commonly associated with the menopause – vaginal dryness, mood swings, bone loss, insomnia, hot flushes and headaches.

PREGNANCY

It may appear inappropriate to list pregnancy under 'prescription medication' but I cannot tell you how many women are told to get pregnant by their doctor – myself included! The idea is similar to that of taking the progesterone-only pill, that a period of rest from menstruation can arrest the symptoms of endometriosis and its progression.

Patients are regularly advised to conceive in the narrow window of time after a surgical procedure in order to boost their chances of reproducing. This is simply not appropriate for some, and there are some women who as a result fear their chances of conceiving are lost outside this allocated time slot. This is simply not the case and further underlines the importance of getting to the root cause of the condition. If you and your partner have planned to have children then this might be a wonderful resolution. But as far as a cure is concerned will it be temporary? Once breastfeeding has finished, symptoms can return and you are left with a rather long-term side effect (in the shape of a child!) unless you adopt lifelong nurturing changes to your lifestyle and diet to maintain hormonal equilibrium.

The length of time for diagnosis averages 11 years. This is partly due to a lack of in-depth knowledge of the disease on the part of GPs but also because of women's acceptance that pain and uncomfortable symptoms are simply part of being a menstruating female. Knowledge amongst GPs on the subject is improving and if women can be more assertive, trusting their own bodies when things do not feel right, diagnosis may be quicker, easier and less emotionally draining.

FINAL WORD

The past decade has seen brilliant progress in research on endometriosis, most especially in surgical procedures. With each discovery we become one step closer to understanding the 'what, why and how' of the condition.

In my view the need for an integrated approach to endometriosis is essential. Research shows that the use of orthodox treatment such as the contraceptive pill, GnRH analogues or danazol, although providing great temporary relief in some women, merely stick a plaster over the condition. Because the actual cause of endometriosis is often not addressed by standard medical practice, the condition and symptoms almost always recur. The side effects of drugs can leave women feeling worse in different ways as well as impact on other areas of their health.

I am not wedded to any particular medical dogma, I am simply a supporter of the get-truly-well philosophy. I strongly support an integration of techniques in managing endometriosis that incorporates investigation into each woman as a whole (body, mind and spirit), including all aspects of her lifestyle. It is an approach that makes use of all appropriate therapies, cherry-picking both conventional and natural practices.

Surgical procedures such as PlasmaJet or laser ablation can create a fabulous starting ground for our body to regain its ability to heal, given the right tools through natural medicine. My aim is to help women acquire knowledge of all the options in treating endometriosis and to respect their own body's brilliant healing capacities. By doing so you can have a profoundly greater ability to make responsible long-lasting choices.

WHY DIET AND LIFESTYLE ARE FUNDAMENTAL TO CONTROLLING ENDOMETRIOSIS 2

With all diseases within the body it has to be a whole-body approach, and when one part of our body is out of balance through disease so too is the rest of it.[1]

Wisdom and now medical research tells us that nutrition is important when dealing with endometriosis. More than important, it is *fundamental*. Feeling like a well-oiled machine may be something you have not felt for a while, or ever, if you have endometriosis.

Research conducted in 2010 for the development of guidelines on the management of endometriosis recognises diet and lifestyle as imperative:

Endometriosis is a common and sometimes debilitating condition for women of reproductive age. A multidisciplinary approach involving a combination of lifestyle modifications, medications, and allied health services should be used to limit the impact of this condition on activities of daily living and fertility.[2]

One particular study undertaken on women who had undergone conservative pelvic surgery for symptomatic moderate/severe endometriosis confirmed the influence of diet in managing endometriosis further.[3] The results showed that nutritional therapy (diet and supplements) was more effective at obtaining relief of pain and improving quality of life than medical hormonal treatment post-surgery.

Until two centuries ago most people in Britain were farmers, who produced their own food. This may seem 'ages ago' but in terms of the physiology of our body, this is merely yesterday. After two centuries of industrialisation our food has undergone some major changes and we've experienced a radical shift in diet. Our bodies are somewhat slow at keeping up with these fast environmental changes and remain relatively primitive. Yet we demand them to keep up with the pace. On the whole our work is less physical, creating a more sedentary existence – regardless of how much we pound the treadmill in the gym, it does not compete with digging for your supper. We consume more processed foods, chemically treated fats and a heady cocktail of artificial additives and toxins from our food than ever before – and we receive fewer nutrients.[4] I use the term 'we' here as however health conscious I am as a nutritional therapist, I too know that the mix of a busy life and a young family mean that at times I fall short of all I need. According to The National Diet and Nutrition Survey published in 2010, at least two thirds of us are not meeting our daily intake of five portions of fruit and vegetables a day. Seeing as '5 a day' is too little to provide for our needs according to some experts, this does not paint a very healthy picture. While consuming toxic and unhealthy substances may feel hard to avoid completely it *should* and *can* be kept to a bare minimum. Our food should feed us not drain us.

In this chapter we will look in more detail at how the links between dietary and lifestyle factors influence the development of endometriosis and pose a threat to your recovery.

DIETARY LINKS
THE LINK WITH NUTRIENT DEFICIENCIES

Nutrient deficiencies come about as a result of not enough of the right food or too much of the wrong food. All systems in the body, both mental and physical, require vitamins and minerals. Our entire being, therefore, can be affected by a lack of nutrients – both physiologically and psychologically. Being low in nutrients does not necessarily equal a diet based on fast food and fizzy drinks. Sometimes it can be that we are eating well but not well enough to provide the specific nutrients we need to heal from a specific condition.

The *Towards a Healthier Britain 2010* report found that as many as 50 per cent of adults were deficient in key nutrients.[5] The researchers revealed that a quarter of women have inadequate intakes of iron and more than 50 per cent lack the antioxidants selenium and magnesium. Antioxidant nutrients are needed to prevent damage to key body cells and their factories. If the antioxidant protection drops because of poor supply, damage to cells can be irretrievable and vital functions such as the hormonal and detoxification systems can be severely compromised, this can lead to diseases such as cancer and other degenerative conditions.

Zinc and magnesium are used up in abundant amounts during states of physical and mental stress; as endometriosis is a state of physical stress, the demand for these nutrients is even greater than normal. During particularly stressful times and during menstruation women can lose up to half their magnesium supply. Women with endometriosis often suffer from heavy bleeding during a period and this significantly reduces their stores of the mineral iron. Without adequate iron stores neurotransmitter function can be affected and this can lead to problems in concentration and general mental acumen, listlessness, low mood and fatigue. It is essential to replenish nutrients through food and, where necessary, supplements, as to manage endometriosis effectively the demand for nutrients is high.

The current system of food production can mean that nutrient deficiencies are common for everyone. Large-scale agriculture and synthetic fertilisers are responsible for a drop in the mineral content of the soil. This view is shared by countless health and environmental experts, such as the Soil Association and Andrew Weil MD.[6] Food production has been speeded up and food quality has deteriorated as a result. Farmers no longer 'raise' cows, pigs or chickens; they fatten them up for the market shelves. The focus of the mass market is now on quantity not quality and consumers can become overweight, undernourished or unwell in the process.

We are also consuming considerably more 'anti-nutrients' from our western existence. Anti-nutrients are those foods and products that actually use up more energy and nutrients from the body than they provide. These include alcohol, sugar, caffeine, smoking, environmental chemicals, heavy metals and medication. Many of today's diseases are caused as much by an excess of anti-nutrients as by a deficiency of nutrients. These not only fail to contribute worthy nutrients, but the body also needs to use high amounts of important antioxidant nutrients just to deal with them. When the supply of anti-nutrients outweighs the store of nutrients inflammation begins and endometriosis can progress.

THE LINK WITH SUGAR

In the past two decades sugar consumption has gone up by 31 per cent, but interestingly sales of sugar in bags has decreased, illustrating the rise in consumption of hidden sugars in foods and confectionery.

Sugar affects the same system within the brain, the opioid system, as nicotine and heroin. Too much glucose in the blood from sugar and unrefined carbohydrates is now widely recognised as harmful to the body and, similar to a drug, the more we have the more our body thinks it need.[7,8] Sugar increases fat, which increases oestrogen production. Sugar, like alcohol, is also an anti-nutrient, depleting the body of valuable vitamins and minerals. Eating foods with sugar causes the pancreas to produce insulin and can encourage an increase in fat cells and, of course, weight gain. Fat cells produce the aromatase enzyme and small amounts of oestrogen. Therefore the more fat cells the more oestrogen is produced. A diet with excess sugar has a link to breast cancer as well.[9,10,11] Too much glucose in the bloodstream also encourages the production of prostaglandin 2 (PGE2), the chemical released by the immune system to cause further inflammation in areas where inflammation already exists, as with endometriosis.

Sugar also reduces the amount of beneficial bacteria that live in the gut. As these bacteria are needed to absorb nutrients from food, a diet high in sugar can quickly lead to poor nutrition and vulnerability to gut complaints. It hinders the absorption of the minerals calcium, chromium and magnesium that are needed for a fully functioning hormonal system and energy production. Chromium and magnesium are also necessary for balancing the amount of glucose in the system; a deficiency of these nutrients can cause a blood sugar condition called hypoglycaemia that can then lead to diabetes. Sugar also blocks the production of anti-inflammatory prostaglandins, thus contributing to the inflammatory nature of endometriosis.

THE LINK WITH THE IMMUNE SYSTEM

The immune system is not only responsible for fighting off colds and flu; it is also essential to the healing process. To aid healing it releases a sophisticated cocktail of chemicals named 'prostaglandins' that either increase or decrease inflammation.

This inflammatory process is a natural protective mechanism to cushion delicate tissue and organs against a threat – something seen as physiologically abnormal and wrong. This process uses a vast amount of nutrients. It then uses these nutrients to heal the damage and regulate the inflammation.

Women with endometriosis do not have strong immune systems. The natural 'killer' cells of the immune system do not work as effectively as they should; endometrial patches that should be regarded as 'invaders', and destroyed by chemicals released by the immune system, are not. Instead they are left intact to roam and migrate to other parts of the body, further provoking inflammation.[12, 13] As the immune system of a woman with endometriosis is usually weaker than the norm it is therefore important to support it in order to control this process.

The hormone system and the immune system require many of the same nutrients: the vitamin B family (especially B6), vitamin C, iron, magnesium, zinc, selenium, the amino acid methionine and vitamins A and E. If any of these are in short supply it can affect both the immune function and the endocrine system.

Sugar can be classed as an anti-nutrient. This means that when eaten, the body uses its store of valuable nutrients such as vitamins A, C and E to deal with sugar. These key nutrients are hightly valuable to the white blood cells of the immune system and can therefore interrupt its functioning if sugar plays a frequent part in your diet.

Stress can dampen down the immune system's ability to function optimally. Under stress the body releases the hormone cortisol. When this is released on a continuous basis (e.g. relentless daily stress such as traffic jams and work strains), it can inhibit the production of progesterone needed for normal equilibrium and the immune system's defence cells.

Results of a major study by the National Institutes of Health and the Endometriosis Association found that women with endometriosis have significantly higher rates of hypothyroidism, fibromyalgia, chronic fatigue syndrome, and auto-immune diseases including rheumatoid arthritis, allergies, asthma and eczema.[14]

THE LINK WITH THE DIGESTIVE SYSTEM

The digestive system is where all nutrients are broken down and prepared for absorption into the bloodstream, so we are as much what we absorb as we are what we eat. If this system is not working well, the ability to produce digestive enzymes to use these nutrients can be weak. Stress may inhibit the effective breakdown of food and the absorption of nutrients, as can low amounts of beneficial bacteria. Without a sufficient amount of the correct nutrients being fed into the bloodstream, hormone production can become erratic.

If you experience symptoms of indigestion, such as bloating, belching, wind, a feeling of being extremely 'full' one to three hours after meals, you are likely to have a low production of digestive enzymes. The approach in this book will address this but if you still experience symptoms after three months you may want to consider a digestive enzyme supplement from one of the companies listed in Further Help.

Without beneficial bacteria, the digestive system's ability to filter what goes into the bloodstream can become affected. Stress (emotional and physical), pesticides, drugs such as the contraceptive pill, antibiotics, antidepressants, or a poor diet can also affect this filter. This might allow particles of food that should be excreted through the gut to be absorbed instead into the bloodstream. The immune system is triggered to attack these foreign particles and inflammation begins. This situation can also encourage food allergies and intolerances as undigested particles of previously innocuous foods are passed into the bloodstream and seen as a threat. The immune system then develops a reaction, which occurs each time that particular food is eaten, until the gut wall is mended by the right nutrients. Studies suggest a link between food intolerances and endometriosis; women with endometriosis appear to have a greater susceptibility to food allergies or intolerances to ordinary foods and chemicals.[15] If you suspect you have food intolerances or an allergy have a look at the Food Intolerance Checker on page 169. If the result proves positive, I think you would benefit from a consultation with a qualified nutritional therapist or from following the elimination diet recommended.

An imbalance in beneficial bacteria can reduce the activity of the enzyme needed to break down excess oestrogen and therefore perpetuate oestrogen dominance.[16] Poor gut flora can allow the naturally present yeast (*Candida albicans*) to proliferate. The excessive growth of *C. albicans* can latch on to the gut wall puncturing small holes and making the situation with the gut filter system worse. An overgrowth of candida cells can upset the fine hormonal balance of the body by attaching themselves to progesterone, rendering it unable to be used and disrupting the balance between oestrogen and progesterone.[17] The majority of women I see in clinic report symptoms of thrush and this indicates an overgrowth of *C. albicans* as a result of low beneficial bacteria. Candida is often treated as a disease; in fact it is a symptom of disease. Candida cannot proliferate if the immune system is strong, so strengthening the immune system diminishes this overgrowth. If you suspect candida is a symptom you are experiencing then use the Have I Got Candida Overgrowth? checker on page 172.

Beneficial bacteria play a primary function in the body's production of B vitamins, a group of vitamins vital for breaking down excess oestrogen. Recent research has confirmed a link between the symptoms of irritable bowel syndrome and endometriosis.[18] The research also showed that a woman is more likely to develop the disease if she has a family history of both endometriosis and irritable bowel syndrome.

THE ROLE OF THE GUT IN INFLAMMATION: This is where the scene of inflammation begins. Picture a digestive environment where over time, and as a result of poor nutrition, the good bacteria have lost the battle against bad bacteria. This is called a state of dysbiosis. If nutrient poor food is added into this environment, bacterial, parasitic or fungal infection begins to take root. These infections wear away parts of the gut's vital 'filter' system, which allows good things into the bloodstream and not so good things out through the rectum. This makes the gut wall 'leak' and previously barred items can escape to float around in the blood. As a result the immune system releases an allergy response to deal with what it sees as a foreign and threatening substance in the blood. Such a response triggers inflammation and can exacerbate the symptoms of endometriosis.

Eighty per cent of the immune system's defence quarters reside in the digestive system and so an unhealthy digestive environment can further weaken an already depleted immune system.

The approach in this book incorporates supporting the gut wall with nourishing foods and supplements. If the digestive system is chronically weakened, I recommend a consultation with an experienced nutritional therapist. To find one in your area, contact the British Association for Applied Nutrition and Nutritional Therapy (BANT), details of which are listed on page 163.

THE LINK WITH THE DETOXIFICATION SYSTEM
We each have our own personal detox system. It is the janitor that never sleeps and labours away night and day clearing unwanted toxins to ensure that hormones are produced and regulated to achieve balance. An excess of hormones such as oestrogen are broken down and removed thereby contributing to hormonal equilibrium. The detox system produces enzymes and amino acids to metabolise fats, proteins and carbohydrates. It stores and supplies nutrients, produces bile for essential fat digestion and regulates blood sugar levels.

> Naturopaths believe that a menstrual period is a means of eliminating toxins and therefore the greater the toxins to excrete, the heavier the period. This is an interesting viewpoint and has correlated with some of the cases I have seen in clinic. Many clients have had a significant reduction in the volume of blood loss once they have lessened their toxic load.

The system manages this effectively until it is presented with too many toxins to handle at any one time. This can have a significant impact on the ability to detoxify or break down the excess of naturally occurring substances in the body, such as oestrogen. If the body is unable to detoxify its own oestrogen, it can result in oestrogen-based conditions such as endometriosis and breast cancer.

An overload of toxins from alcohol, drugs, fatty foods, highly refined foods such as sugar, medicines such as the pill, environmental toxins from fumes, pesticides and xeno-oestrogens can overload the liver if there are not the right nutritional resources to deal with them. If these toxins block the smooth elimination process, the liver can begin to suffer. Blood sugar levels begin to fluctuate resulting in tiredness, and craving for stimulants and sugary foods. Hormone balance is disrupted and symptoms of premenstrual syndrome, night sweats, hair loss, increased pain or disrupted cycles can be experienced.

The skin, another major detoxification organ, can suffer too. Waste products are removed through the skin's pores in sweat and the skin's 'breath'. If this exit becomes blocked, or there is a queue at the exit, the condition of the skin, hair and nails can suffer. These are clear warning signs that nutrients are low and toxin levels are high.

The chemical load in the environment is increasing and adds additional work for the body to process. There are now over 300 environmental chemicals around us on a daily basis.[19]

LIFESTYLE LINKS
THE LINK WITH ENVIRONMENTAL TOXINS
Every day a sea of potentially hormone-disrupting toxins surrounds us. They come from the air that we breathe, the packaging of our food, the water we drink, the chemicals we put on our skin, detergents, household cleaning products, artificial fragrances in perfumes and air fresheners, pesticides and exhaust fumes. You get the picture.

It goes without saying that the body does not want these, nor does it need them. On top of all this, diets often do not provide the nutrients the body needs in the right quantities to deal with this onslaught effectively.

Sixty per cent of these chemicals are absorbed and collected in the body through the skin. Think about the principle of an HRT or nicorette patch to understand how effectively they are absorbed. If you live in an urban or semi-urban environment, your body will be subject to an even greater bombardment.

Some of the unwanted chemicals have a similar physical structure to that of natural oestrogen and it is essential that women with endometriosis avoid these. These chemicals are known as 'xeno-oestrogens'. When inside the body they can fox the system into thinking they are genuine, natural structures of oestrogen. Tricked, the body allows these chemical 'cowboys' to connect with the cells that communicate with oestrogen and interfere with the balance. They have been termed oestrogen 'mimics' and you can understand why. For a body that already has a hormonal imbalance such as endometriosis these chemicals pose a real threat.[20]

A xeno-oestrogen that has received a lot of interest is the chemical dioxin. Studies demonstrate that chronic exposure to dioxin is directly linked to the development and progression of endometriosis.[21,22] Dioxins also appear to block the body's production and use of progesterone, upsetting the balance between oestrogen and progesterone and perpetuating oestrogen dominance.[23,24] Dioxins are known to suppress the immune system.[25,26] According to research,[27,28] including that done by The Environmental Protection Agency in the United States, the 'body burdens of, and exposure to, dioxins are already at levels which affect our health'.[29] One of the specific health concerns listed by this agency was 'the higher probability of experiencing endometriosis and the reduced ability to withstand immunological challenge'.

I have had the privilege of working with a leading medical expert on endometriosis, Professor Chris Sutton (pioneer of the laser technology for treating endometriosis in the UK), who is similarly convinced of the detrimental influence artificial substances such as dioxins have on the development and progression of the condition.

Dioxins are by-products of industrial incineration and combustion. They are also produced by the manufacturing of chlorine-containing pesticides, wood preservatives and paper. Dioxins persist in the environment for years and accumulate in the fat of farm animals that eat contaminated feed or water. Linked by some studies to endometriosis, these toxins appear to disrupt hormone function, causing imbalances.

According to a report by the World Health Organization, the highest concentration of dioxin in breast milk in the world is in Belgium.[30] The country's southern industrial corridor has extremely high amounts of environmental dioxin and polychlorinated biphenyl (PCB) pollution. It also has the highest concentration of cases of advanced, deep infiltrating endometriosis.[31] Some experts think this is hard evidence that environmental exposure to such pollutants is a contributory factor in the development and progression of endometriosis. Dioxins have also been shown to exert a disruptive effect on the beneficial gut flora.[32]

Xeno-estrogens are almost ubiquitous in modern food production, and what is worse they most often come as a cocktail with other separately harmful toxins. This cocktail is in the pesticides sprayed on crops, in the plastic packaging for salads, ready meals and vegetables and feminine hygiene and household products. Animals consume pesticide and herbicide-laden food, we eat the meat and by-products such as dairy, and the cycle continues. What frustrates me endlessly about the companies that use and produce these chemical toxins is their defence that the amount of the toxin that would need to be ingested to cause harm is unachievably high in 'normal' living. But this is when the chemical is in isolation. What happens when we are unwittingly exposed to an environmental stew of different chemicals? In his book, *Our Stolen Future*, Dr Theo Colborn found the cocktail of chemicals that people in the 'west' are exposed to not only interferes with hormonal health but actually changes the structure of our genes a thousand times more than when exposed to one chemical in isolation. In other words xeno-oestrogens bio-magnify. This means that they build up in the body's fatty tissue over time, gathering a collective strength. Considering it can take up to seven years to rid the body of just half the amount of the accumulated xeno-oestrogens in the system, it is essential that women with endometriosis reduce their intake in the first place.[34,35]

Prenatal exposure to xeno-oestrogens is an important area of developing research. The neonatal and prenatal stages are critical in terms of development and sensitivity to toxic chemicals.[36] It is possible for the mother to excrete half of her accumulated xeno-oestrogens in breast milk during lactation.[37] Many health professionals have a growing concern over this and the development of endometriosis and research is needed.

Many processed foods come in packaging ready for heating. Heat increases the chance of the food absorbing the toxins within the packaging. These foods also tend to contain fats that encourage the absorption of these chemical products. Pre-prepared foods such as fruit and vegetables are often packed in aluminium and plastic, which significantly add to the toxic load. Drinks packaged in cans or plastic bottles can also absorb the chemicals in their packaging and therefore glass bottles are preferable.

The health concerns of these pollutants are, in fact, a threat to *any* woman of *any* age. For more information on how and why to avoid these chemicals please refer to appendix 6 Keeping Clean and Green on page 174.

SMOKING

It goes without saying that smoking is not going to benefit any health condition but this is especially true in women with endometriosis. It is important for smokers (social smokers or full time!) to make their choice an educated one. Smoking is a significant anti-nutrient. Not only does it rob the body of vitamin C (25mg per cigarette), calcium and the whole B vitamin family but it also fills the body with high levels of the heavy toxic metal cadmium (see 'Heavy metals' section). Cadmium prevents the body using zinc properly, a key mineral for a healthy menstrual cycle. Tobacco exposure is related to reduced ovarian function.[39] The picture is not a pretty one and I cannot impress on you enough that quitting smoking will give you a very healthy reward.

If you have the wisdom to quit, take a good antioxidant combination supplement. This will not only work to replace your lost nutrients, it will also support repair of the damage caused by smoking and help to reduce the cravings. Acupuncture also has a good track record for helping you to stub them out, as has hypnotherapy. As with all changes of habit, you have to fully want to give up in order for it to work.

WATER

Without water we cannot survive, so it may seem strange having water in this section. Water replenishes, cleanses and regenerates the kidneys, adrenals and liver. It is the most important feature in any healthy existence and particularly for any cleansing, detoxification diet. But here is the quandary. Standard methods of purifying water by the regional water boards remove bugs but leave behind dissolved chemicals, of which there are estimated to be approximately 60,000. In attempts to clean the water aluminium and chlorine are added; toxic in their own right they also have the capacity to combine with other compounds to create havoc with the hormonal system. Sales of bottled water have shot through the roof in the past five years as this knowledge has become more widespread. We will look at the role of pure water in subsequent chapters.

THE CONTRACEPTIVE PILL AND MEDICATION

The contraceptive pill is one of the most common forms of treatment for endometriosis but I would urge you to think twice about this treatment. The pill can cause a number of nutrient deficiencies, including vitamins B1, B2, B6, B12, C and E and the important mineral zinc.[40,41]

It can also reduce progesterone that in turn can lead to oestrogen dominance.[42] This can exacerbate the symptoms of endometriosis, as well as other conditions such as polycystic ovary syndrome (PCOS).

Oestrogens present in the contraceptive pill can affect insulin metabolism and therefore upset a healthy blood sugar balance.[43] Older brands of the pill are potentially the worst culprits, creating a soar in oestrogen levels. If the body is already receiving a bulk of xeno-oestrogens from the environment, adding more through the pill creates further imbalance.

Research has provided good evidence to suggest that young women who take the contraceptive pill run a higher risk of developing premenopausal breast cancer.[44,45,46]

If you choose to go on or stay on the pill, you need to be extra-vigilant about your diet and reducing your chemical load. It is advisable take a good multi-nutrient supplement.

Taking steroids (sometimes prescribed for reducing inflammation associated with severe endometriosis) over a long period of time can seriously limit the amount of B vitamins that are needed to synthesise energy from food and remove excess oestrogen. Regular (2–3 times per month for example) use of non-steroidal anti-inflammatory drugs (NSAIDS) such as ibuprofen decreases the beneficial bacteria in the gut. They can affect the breakdown of oestrogen and the absorption of nutrients from food, as well as affecting the toxic load with which the liver must deal.

Antidepressants may also disrupt the gut flora and liver enzyme function preventing the absorption of nutrients and perpetuating the symptoms of endometriosis.

HEAVY METALS OR METALLOESTROGENS

Metalloestrogens are a new class of hormone disrupters made up of the environmental heavy metals lead, mercury, cadmium and aluminium. These disturb hormonal balance by getting into cells and tissues. This disrupts the normal function of the neurotransmitters within the brain, the nervous system, the hormonal system and the immune system.[47] This will impair protection against disease and increase the body's sensitivity to stress. The heavy metals are stored in body fat to protect the organs by removing the metals from the circulation. But they are also stored in the fatty tissue within our hormone-producing glands.

The results of an investigation into hormone-related disease and pesticides indicated that women with hormone irregularities or specific fertility disorders might have been influenced by heavy metals found in non-organic food and pesticides.[48]

FINAL WORD

Food is a powerful medicine that has a huge impact on the chemical processes in the body. Many of the symptoms of endometriosis can be improved by what we eat and, just as importantly, what we don't eat. I have seen it time and time again in my clinic. Healthy changes can boost your immune system, improve energy, reduce pain associated with inflammation, balance your menstrual cycle, and improve the chances of fertility, to name just a few. But the most important thing is that it is *you* that can make these changes happen.

Even after years of neglect, it is never too late to change your lifestyle and significantly improve your health. The body has an amazing ability to heal itself if given the chance and by acquiring healthier habits you can actually rejuvenate it.

PART 2

TAKE CONTROL: THE NURTURE DIET FOR MANAGING YOUR ENDOMETRIOSIS NATURALLY AND SUSTAINABLY

EATING CONSCIOUSLY 3

Before following the Nurture Diet for the first time I recommend that you complete the Kickstart Cleanse programme outlined in Chapter 6. This will give your body the perfect introduction to healing. By initiating the cleansing and repairing of major detoxification organs through nutrition you will also set up some fundamental, positive healthy eating habits. Eating consciously is building on those deliberate changes so I advise that you read and understand this chapter first. We will look at the need to continue supporting hormonal equilibrium so you can manage the symptoms of endometriosis.

This chapter, in fact this entire book, is not designed to arm you with more reasons to feel guilt around food (we women are very good at that). Rather it is to inform so that you can make sound, intelligent choices to eat and live in a nurturing way that helps you to control the role endometriosis plays in your life. It is not about giving yourself a mental thrashing for eating a burger and chips or drinking a glass too much of wine. The Nurture Diet has been tailored to fit in with everyday life. I want you to be able to follow this way of living within the parameters of your normal existence. I want you to have the opportunity to adopt some positive, long-term changes so that *you* can control how you feel as much as you can on a day-to-day basis.

Eating 'healthily' or 'a balanced diet' are key phrases nowadays but what exactly do they mean? The fact is that the terms 'balanced diet' and 'healthy eating' can be misleading. Yes there are the fundamental rules of healthy eating that we are told about by government initiatives and magazines for example. But these are building blocks. They are not the one-stop-shop answer for many people. Endometriosis is a key example of that. It may be okay for your friend Carol to dig into a bowl of pasta with fresh tomato sauce but that might not be healthy for *you*. By understanding your condition and informing yourself of what your body needs and doesn't need you can find a healthy and individual way of eating and living that works especially for you. Just because we cannot see endometriosis does not mean we can ignore it.

Food is there to nourish us. Eating healthily means experimenting with your cooking skills and with ingredients, varying the foods you eat, packing meals with exciting vegetables rather than bland old peas on the side of the plate. Many of us cook the same old worn-out recipes for ease and convenience at the end of a tiring day. This can mean we do not have full access to the range of nutrients our body needs, and mealtimes are not exciting to our senses.

Add to this the fact that the majority of us cook when we are already hungry and tired, a lethal combination: we may be tempted to cook food in portions that are too big for our needs. We choose easy options, foods that do not nurture us nutritionally, and we often end up eating late (less than three hours before going to bed).

Try to eat seasonal fruits or vegetables you may not even recognise; if you don't know what to do with them indulge in some specialist recipe books. I have listed some of my favourites in the Further Help section. Respecting your health and body also means not 'stuffing your face' when you are hungry, but stopping when you are 80 per cent full to avoid overloading and straining your digestive system. Override your appetite requirements at your hips' and your health's peril.

Managing endometriosis naturally is about supporting the immune system to reduce inflammation and bring the disrupted hormone balance back into equilibrium. A diet to support this approach is largely based on whole-foods and avoiding excess fats and chemicals. A nutrient-rich diet such as suggested in this chapter can have a positive effect on all aspects of health including digestive well-being, optimum immune function and maintaining a healthy weight. As I have discussed in Chapter 2, certain foods and environmental factors affect the amount of oestrogen our body encounters and limiting these is key.

Lifestyle habits such as stress (yes this is a habit) and a lack of exercise can affect the body's ability to deal with both physical and mental symptoms of endometriosis and so, in Chapter 4, we will also be looking at these in more detail.

The quality of the food is vital. In our contemporary way of living, the healthy choice is not always the easy option so this chapter aims to help you make the most convenient and healthy choices that also fit in with your life. Eating and living naturally means that you nourish your body and your mind in a way that is lasting.

After just one month of following this diet you should begin to notice a significant improvement in your general well-being such as enhanced energy levels or better skin condition for example, as well as a clear decrease in the symptoms of your endometriosis.

BECOME SLOW AND UNREFINED

The more refined a food is, the less nutrition it will provide. Carbohydrates can either be refined or unrefined, or to put it more aptly, fast or slow. If refined or fast, they provide a concentration of quick-releasing sugars that rush into our bloodstream, causing a surge of glucose. This instructs the body to release the hormone insulin to carry away the excess glucose to store in muscle and fat cells. The resulting physical effects are a surge of energy followed by a crash. We are left feeling exhausted and hormone imbalance is exacerbated. We then find ourselves craving sugar-loaded foods or stimulants, such as caffeine, to give us back our energy, and the cycle continues.

Eating unrefined or slow carbohydrates, however, ensures that a slow and consistent supply of glucose is leaked into the bloodstream. This provides the body with the correct amount of fuel for the energy it needs, and stabilises blood sugar balance. Unrefined carbohydrates include wholegrain rice, wholewheat, quinoa, barley, rye and oats. Research has shown us that slow carbohydrates in wholegrain products also stimulate the production of serotonin, a neurotransmitter that creates a sense of well-being, and improves concentration and sleep.[1]

Some health professionals recommend following a diet based on the glycaemic index, which dictates your eating habits by the extent to which foods raise blood sugar levels after eating. The glycemic index (GI) is a ranking of carbohydrates on a scale from 0 to 100. Foods with a high GI are those which are rapidly digested and absorbed and result in marked fluctuations in blood sugar levels. Low-GI foods, by virtue of their slow digestion and absorption, produce gradual rises in blood sugar and insulin levels, and have proven benefits for health. Although a good starting point it is by no means the complete answer. By default this rules out some of the less healthy foods such as confectionery or white flour products but it also rules out some foods that do bring health benefits. For example, foods indicated as acceptable to eat are ice cream and sausages. Bananas and baked potatoes however are seen to have a 'high glycaemic index', foods to limit or avoid. From this point of view I find this approach simplistic and misleading. Adding some protein to a carbohydrate food slows the speed at which the glucose is released into the bloodstream – so it becomes more of a drip, drip than a flood. Chopping some banana, adding it to Greek yogurt and sprinkling on some seeds, or filling your baked potato with hummus and avocado is, to me, a whole lot more nutritious than some sausages and a bowl of ice cream.

Look for sugar in packaged foods; the higher up the ingredients list it is, the higher the content. Don't replace sugar with sweeteners, these are just as toxic and evidence suggests they could be carcinogenic.[2,3] It is a good idea to reduce a 'sweet tooth' but in those moments when fruit just won't cut it, try some honey (local or Manuka/active honey preferably) on a cracker or some yogurt. Or have a little bit of dark chocolate, 70 per cent cocoa solids and above, maybe even with some dried fruit inside. Although dark chocolate contains caffeine, its benefits outweigh its negatives if eaten in small amounts because it contains a high amount of antioxidant nutrients used to repair and protect areas of tissue damage. Dried fruit also contains high amounts of natural fast-releasing sugars called fructose, but the breakdown is slowed, becoming a 'slow carbohydrate' because of the amount of fibre they contain.

AVOID: Refined carbohydrates include sugar and all its products – cakes, confectionery and biscuits – and white flour products.

BOOST: Wholemeal grains such as quinoa, barley, wholegrain rice and oatbran.

TIP: Sweeten foods with honey, maple syrup or dried fruit rather than sugar.

BULK UP

Forms of fibre include the wholegrains oats, barley, quinoa, rye, millet and buckwheat, and fruit and vegetables are primary sources too.

Research shows women who ate green vegetables 13 times or more per week (roughly twice a day) were 70 per cent less likely to have endometriosis than those who ate green vegetables less than six times per week.[4] Women who ate fresh fruit 14 times or more per week (at least twice a day) were 40 per cent less likely to have endometriosis than those who ate fruit and vegetables less than six times per week. These studies cement the proposition that eating a variety of fresh fruit and vegetables (at least 5 of each) everyday can have a contributory effect on reducing your symptoms of endometriosis.

Nearly all fruits, vegetables and pulses, such as lentils and chickpeas, are also alkaline-forming. It is thought that if your blood is more 'acidic', you have a greater propensity to inflammation.[5] As this nurturing lifestyle is abundant with alkaline-forming foods this will be addressed by default.

In case you didn't know already, fruit and vegetables are jam-packed with nutrients, phytonutrients to be exact ('phyto' meaning plant and 'nutrients' meaning vitamins and minerals). What is more, the colour found in fruits and vegetables is the result of a group of nutrients that have a potent ability to repair damage. Known as carotenoids and flavanoids these natural nutrients boost the immune system and supply the tools for repair. The key is in variety so get as much colour as you can on your plate each day. As carotenoids and flavanoids are all found naturally within the foods, they can be used very easily by our bodies with less work and great benefits.

Vegetable and fruit fibre encourages the growth of friendly gut bacteria that support the digestive system and reduce the reabsorption of oestrogen into the bloodstream by clearing hormone debris.

Dark green leafy vegetables contain substances called 'phyto-oestrogens' that can protect against oestrogen-related diseases such as endometriosis. Phyto-oestrogens do this by binding to excess oestrogen in the gut and thereby encouraging its elimination.[6] The cabbage family, including cabbages, broccoli, kale, bok choy, cauliflower, Brussels sprouts and radicchio, contain substances called 'indoles' that can encourage the breakdown of oestrogen.

Lemons are wonderful at alkalising the body's tissues and reducing inflammation. Use on salads, pasta and in warm water with ginger.

If you cannot buy fresh vegetables, frozen are better than tinned, as freezing often takes place immediately after picking and therefore retains many of their nutrients (nutrients start to deplete once picked).

BOOST: Vegetables and fruits high in healthy phytonutrients include apples, avocado, squash, broccoli, cherries, pineapple, peppers, tomatoes, spinach, carrots, sweet potato, blueberries, oranges, kale, cauliflower and aubergine (in Traditional Chinese Medicine (TCM) this plant is great for circulation encouraging the removal of old blood and delivery of new fresh blood).

TIP: Home bean and seed sprouters are an excellent way to get a boost of phytonutrients that don't cost the earth. You can sprout just about anything: sunflower, broccoli, wheatgrass, mung beans or chickpeas. They are full of goodness and easy to maintain.

STABILISE YOUR HORMONES WITH PLANTS

Phyto-oestrogens are plant compounds that mimic a weak version of oestrogen in the body. All cells have oestrogen receptors that act like a lock, with oestrogen as the key for certain processes. Phyto-oestrogens can block this lock and key system thereby preventing the activation of excess oestrogen. Where there is not enough oestrogen present (such as after the menopause) the phyto-oestrogens can slot into the 'lock' in the cell and exert mild oestrogenic properties helping to reduce symptoms when oestrogen is too low, such as poor bone density. These foods also support the liver in breaking down excess oestrogen.

BOOST: Phyto-oestrogen rich foods include pulses, chickpeas, lentils and soya. Products of phyto-oestrogen foods include tofu, tempeh, soya milk, hummus, lentils (curries such as dhal for example) and baked beans (although watch out for the brands that contain sugar).

TIP: The above foods may cause flatulence but eating only a small amount every day will reduce the 'wind' effect! As the intestines get used to these foods being in the diet more often, the wind will settle too.

GET FRIENDLY WITH YOUR GUT

The absorption of nutrients from food happens in the gastrointestinal tract. The health of your digestive system is therefore key to the management of conditions such as endometriosis. Yogurt (cow's, goat's, sheep's or soya) contains beneficial bacteria, mainly *Lactobacillus acidophilus*, which reduces the production of a substance called beta-glucuronidase. This is the enzyme that remakes oestrogen in the gut from hormone debris and encourages it to be reabsorbed into the bloodstream. Beneficial bacteria also support immune function (up to 70 per cent of the immune system is in the gut). Always look for yogurt with *live* bacteria in. If you need to avoid dairy products for health or through choice then consider a probiotic supplement from a reputable supplement company as listed in Useful Contacts.

BOOST: Live, plain organic yogurt or dairy-free alternatives (avoid those with sugar in them – most flavoured versions have sugar added) and sauerkraut.

TIP: Use yogurt to make dressings and sauces.

ENSURE YOUR FATS ARE ESSENTIAL

While saturated fats encourage the inflammatory process that may exacerbate endometriosis, essential fats found in nuts, seeds and fish such as salmon, kippers, tuna (fresh) and sardines reduce inflammation. These fatty acids are called omega 3 and are the foundation stones in the production of the anti-inflammatory prostaglandins, PGE1 and PGE3. These prostaglandins are made in the body continuously, 24 hours a day, 7 days a week, as they have a very short lifespan. This means the body is reliant on us to ingest a regular supply of omega 3 to produce them. The function of the immune system is dependent upon an adequate amount of these essential fatty acids to stay strong. Look for fish from reliable sources to reduce exposure to unwanted chemicals found in the seas (for more information see the Sustainable Fish Guide in the Useful Contacts section, page 164). It is important to note that production of anti-inflammatory PGE1 and PGE3 is blocked by processed oils and margarines, as well as white flour, sugar, excessive animal fats, alcohol, poor nutrition and stress. Keeping these to a minimum is vital to reduce inflammation.

Another group of fatty acids are the omega 6 fatty acids. They are essential but found in abundance in our western diets, so we do not need to concentrate on incorporating these. The ratio between omega 3 and omega 6 is important and so including a good supply of omega 3 in your diet is important to keep this ratio balanced.

BOOST: Oily fish such as mackerel, fresh tuna, sardines, salmon, brazil nuts, walnuts, hazelnuts, pecans, sunflower seeds, pumpkin seeds, hemp seeds, cold-pressed nut and seed oils and avocado.

TIP: Try to eat a small handful of mixed nuts and seeds (whole or ground), which you can add to food such as salads or stir-fries, or eat as a snack but chewed well. You can slow roast them at a low temperature (150–180°C) for 15 minutes. Eat oily fish up to three times per week.

GET LEAN

Eat small amounts of protein with *every* meal. Good quality, lean sources of protein help to maintain blood sugar balance needed for energy, and give your body an even supply of the amino acids needed to build and repair cells, plus manufacture and maintain balanced hormones. By eating lean protein with a 'slow' carbohydrate you are providing your body with the tools for its 'well-being factory'.

BOOST: Choose lean sources of protein such as fish, chicken, turkey, eggs or pulses such as lentils, chickpeas, nuts and seeds. Include health-promoting dairy products such as yogurt from cow's milk or goat's/sheep's milk if preferable for taste or due to a cow's milk intolerance.

TIP: Whilst I do not advocate tinned vegetables, pulses are an exception. Try throwing tinned pulses such as chickpeas, lentils or borlotti beans into your salads, soups, stir-fries or tagines for example. For a list of sustainable fish species to enjoy, see the Useful Contacts section on page 164.

GO ORGANIC

Organic farming in the UK is governed by strict standards and involves avoiding the use of unhealthy pesticides and fertilisers not on an approved list. This is a really good thing as many of these chemicals are hormone-disrupters. Organic meat comes from animals that are raised in natural conditions, on organically farmed land and are not treated routinely with antibiotics.

Artificial oestrogen-like hormones are fed to non-organic cattle to keep the cows in milk and to fatten them up. This passes directly into us through their by-products. Conversely, meat from organically reared animals is nutrient rich because of their healthier diet and lifestyle and, for me, it is preferable to know that the animal had a natural existence rather than a factory style one. Some research suggests that if the animal is happy this can even improve the taste as stress can toughen the meat.

We have to live in the real world, so eating organic exclusively is pretty hard. Choosing organic dairy foods and meat, though, can make a significant difference to the amount of environmental chemicals you put into your body. Organic products are more expensive but most of them are worth the extra pennies. Where possible, organic fruit and veg that doesn't have a peel is also worth buying. Going organic also means you will tend to eat more seasonal food too.

'Organic' is now a buzzword that, in commercial terms, can generate greater profit for supermarkets. Organic standards vary from country to country and so I would feel inclined to trust an organic food from the UK more than one from other sources. Look for certification from well-respected organisations such as the Soil Association. For more information on trustworthy organic organisations around the world contact the International Federation of Organic Agriculture movements listed in Further Help. Some companies also produce organic 'convenience' foods. Although they no doubt contain organic produce, you can sometimes be misled into thinking it is a health food. In fact extra salt or sugar can be added so still check the labels.

On the whole buying organic is most important when it comes to dairy products and meat. These are the areas of non-organic food production that are the most heavily consumed and therefore are more vulnerable to 'chemical intervention' to ensure that supply meets demand. If your budget will not stretch to buying the full organic range, do make a priority in your budget for these products.

BOOST: The following will reduce your exposure to environmental toxins greatly: buy loose vegetables and fruit, wash salads in filtered water yourself, eat organic meat and dairy and buy local where possible.

TIP: Try buying one extra organic product each week to get into the habit.

SATURATED FATS

Although we do need a little saturated fat in our diets it is far from ideal to have too much. A small amount of saturated fat is needed as is a small portion of red meat (about twice a week is optimum) and should be enjoyed as part of a healthy diet. I am a big fan of good, organic butter and also like to roast my potatoes in goose fat, but I am mindful of not tipping the balance.

Dairy produce and red meat are rich sources of saturated fat and contain a substance called arachadonic acid. In excess arachadonic acid triggers the production of PGE2. As we have discussed before this is a highly inflammatory prostaglandin that can cause swelling and pain, associated endometrial cramps and the spread of endometrial tissue.[7]

A recent study has shown women who eat a diet high in red meat may be at increased risk of endometriosis.[8] The study showed that women who ate beef or other red meat seven times a week or more were 100 per cent more likely to have endometriosis than women who ate red meat three times a week or less. Women who ate ham three or more times per week were 80 per cent more likely to have endometriosis than those who ate it less than once per week. The same study also demonstrated that eating a diet high in fruit and vegetables may reduce the risk of the condition.

When the urge for a burger occurs I see nothing wrong with indulging yourself once in a while. Just make sure it is of high quality and includes a side salad!

Remember that pork, and its products such as ham, sausagemeat and bacon, is a red meat too. Endometriosis sufferer or not, limit red meat intake to preferably twice, but a maximum of three, times a week. If you are concerned about missing the iron levels in meat, there are many alternative sources of these nutrients.

Boost: For an iron boost make sure you include plenty of spinach, pumpkin seeds, parsley, almonds, prunes, cashews, raisins, walnuts and pecan nuts in your diet. Nuts and dried fruit are great as a mixture to use as a snack to dip into during the day or to add to salads or cereals.

TRANS FATS

Trans fats are the result of hydrogenated, processed or heavily refined oils. They have received a lot of negative press in recent years and I am pleased to say are being removed from the shelves of the more conscientious food chains. They are used to preserve foods and have a morphed chemical structure that interrupts the function of cells and can weaken defences as well as encourage inflammation. These weakened defences are thought to be the reason that trans fats can encourage the implantation of endometrial patches and they have also been associated with breast cancer.[9] Trans fats can be found in fried foods including some crisps and frozen chips.

In my mind margarines should be banned for all eternity. Most are made by a process called hydrogenation and mix cheap fats with particles of metal. Despite various health claims to lower this and boost that, I passionately believe that it is better for your well-being to enjoy a little butter in your life. Keep it in a cool place to avoid it going rancid and becoming a trans fat because heat changes the chemical structure of fats turning them into a trans fat.

TIP: Heating oils can change their chemical structure to trans oils, 180°C for olive oil for example. Rapeseed oil has a higher 'turning' point and so maintains its omega 3 and 6 content at higher temperatures. Vegetable oil and butter do not become trans fats when heated but are still not ideal. The answer is to limit frying food in fat to a minimum and consider options such as steam frying by adding a tablespoon of water into a hot pan, using the resultant steam to cook with. You may need to add more water as you cook, and make sure the pan stays hot otherwise the food will go soggy. Although this method uses a high heat it is for a much shorter amount of time and therefore still retains a good amount of the food's nutrient content.

ALCOHOL

Alcohol interferes with hormonal health. Too much isn't a good idea for several reasons. Firstly, it provides zero nutrients and a lot of empty calories. It uses up stores of nutrients including the important hormonal regulators, the B vitamin group, magnesium and zinc. A large glass of wine contains a high amount of sugar, which can also lead to weight gain. Resulting fat cells produce oestrogen, which contributes to oestrogen dominance. The sugar content of alcohol can also bring about rapidly rising glucose levels in the bloodstream, followed by a sudden drop. This yo-yo effect can leave the body mentally and physically tired. As the liver is the only organ that can metabolise alcohol, an excess consumption can interfere with normal functioning, making this organ less able to dispose of excess oestrogen. Some clients have reported symptoms of endometriosis such as pain in the pelvic region (or where their patches of endometriosis are located) the morning after a 'heavy night' and this is probably why.

There is no doubt that the detrimental effects of alcohol are directly related to the amount you drink, and the time period over which you drink it. Drink consciously and allow it to be a friend and not a foe. Enjoying alcohol in moderation is a fabulous pleasure in life and maintaining a balanced relationship with it is important. Red wine exerts health benefits in small amounts (one glass every other day maximum). A tipple of vino rosso would seem to be the drink of choice although don't be shy with the pennies as cheaper red wines can have a toxic mould, ochratoxin, which can induce allergy-like reactions such as aching in the muscles or joints that can be worse in areas where inflammation exists already, which is the case with endometriosis. White wine contains high amounts of histamine – a chemical that can set off allergic reactions in those with atopic allergies, so watch out for this if you have hayfever, eczema or asthma. Beer and grain-based products tend to have gluten in them and are best avoided by anyone with a gluten intolerance. As research is increasingly suggesting that there is a

BOOST: Increase your intake of fruit or vegetable juices instead of alcohol. My tipple is a virgin Bloody Mary.

TIP: When you do drink alcohol make it a quality wine or spirit and don't drink on an empty stomach – a good excuse to sample the healthy canapés.

link between gluten and endometriosis I suggest these products are limited, if not avoided.

Let's not forget the influential fact of waking up feeling a bit better on Sunday mornings as well!

CAFFEINE

In 1998 a study conducted on a group of women with endometriosis asked the participants to eliminate caffeine from their diet and to supplement it with essential fatty acids for a period of time.[10] The results showed significantly beneficial results with a reduction in pain and symptoms of endometriosis, such as fatigue.

Caffeine is found in coffee beans, tea leaves, cocoa beans, energy boosting type drinks, cola and guarana. It can also be found in medications such as hangover and cold remedies so watch out for this too. I know how difficult cutting out a good café latte or cappuccino can be – it was the hardest thing for me to do – but read on and look at the evidence. Caffeine has a diuretic effect and so again acts as an anti-nutrient, blocking or taking away vital stores of vitamins and minerals, such as iron, that are essential for a healthy hormone balance. Like sugar, caffeine overstimulates the adrenal glands responsible for the effective management of stress and the regulation of energy and sleep. Persistent and chronic caffeine consumption weakens the adrenal system and a cycle develops where you need greater and greater amounts to get an effect. You may also suffer headaches or irritability if you don't get your 'shot'. Some women and men drink caffeine because they think it curbs their appetite – this may be the case temporarily, like smoking, but once the blood sugar levels drop again they will find themselves shaky, hungry and craving another immediate fix in the form of more caffeine, a cigarette or carbohydrates and sugar. Caffeine also requires the liver to remove it, which can take the liver's attention away from breaking down excess oestrogen levels. Drinking more than two cups of coffee per day has been linked to endometriosis.[11] Remember too that the frothy versions you can buy often have more than the one shot of strong coffee in them. If the idea of a caffeine-free existence fills you with horror then one cup of green tea a day is not only tasty to drink (try with a squeeze of lemon or a small amount of honey), it has also been shown to exert beneficial health properties by providing antioxidants that work in the body to combat areas of damage.

BOOST: Experiment with herbal teas. There are some fabulous loose teas available that are worth considering for example: for digestion: peppermint, fennel, ginger, cinnamon; as a calmative: verbena, camomile, valerian, lemon balm; as a muscle relaxant: raspberry leaf (avoid if pregnant).

TIP: Rosemary contains a substance called indole that encourages the breakdown of oestrogen. You can make a tea with rosemary sprigs and drink three times per day. Herbal teas also have the benefit of contributing to your daily intake of water.

Food allergies and intolerances

It is now accepted that whilst certain foods can cure you, others can equally make you unwell. Food allergies and intolerances to ordinary foods are growing more common among the general population but there is a body of evidence developing that suggests that women with endometriosis suffer higher rates of food allergies and intolerances because of the condition.[12]

These reactions are often to common foodstuffs and everyday environmental chemicals. The cause is likely to be that both the immune system and optimum gut function can be weakened in women with endometriosis. Food intolerances and allergies require a damaged digestive 'filter' in order to occur, such as where particles have leaked through the gut into the bloodstream, or there are insufficient digestive enzymes to break the food down in the first place. What may also be contributing to this is the rise in the use of environmental chemicals and the artificial manipulation of foods (think the 'refining' process, GM crops etc.), which could be adding further strain to our immune defences. Our busy and often stressful way of life may also limit the amount of nutritionally rich food we eat, as well as placing a higher demand for nutrients in order to cope with the pace. All in all we have a melting pot of contributory factors that can make food allergies and intolerances an even greater risk to women with endometriosis.

With allergies, the immune system releases the chemicals IgA or IgE into the bloodstream in response to what it sees as a foreign substance, and to meet any threat. Depending on whether IgA or IgE is released you could experience a potentially fatal anaphylactic shock or another physical response such as an immediate rash or swelling. Allergies are very different to intolerances and all allergies are potentially life threatening if not given the necessary attention.

In food intolerances the reaction is subtler and can remain hidden for hours or days. Food intolerances can make us feel tired and achy, and suffer from headaches, digestive complaints such as bloating, weight gain, skin conditions such as eczema and sometimes even depression (possibly partly to do with feeling the array of other symptoms). Food intolerances are harder to detect and the symptoms can creep up on you so slyly that you may accept it as normal living: 'I feel tired today'. What happens in this situation is that you continue to eat the trigger food and the immune system continues to send out chemicals to attack it (this time a substance called IgG). Frequently this process turns into a cycle by producing a craving for the food in question. The immune system can then become tired, using up much of its defending army which is needed to prevent other invaders. Food intolerances can therefore weaken your immune defences over time and actively increase your vulnerability to infections in places such as the sinuses, throat, ears and tonsils. They also actively perpetuate inflammation elsewhere in the body; not good news for endometriosis sufferers. An intolerance can be temporary if given the right nutritonal attention, however, it is very unlikely that an adult will outgrow a true food allergy.

The most common food intolerances are to cow's milk products (cheese, milk, cream), food preservatives and colourings such as Azo dyes (Tartrazine) and Non-azo dyes (erythrocine) or Nitrates and Nitrites (E 249 – E 252), which give meat a pink colour to look more attractive and are found in bacon, salami and frankfurters; wheat (bread, cakes, biscuits, pastries, pastas), eggs, citrus fruits and foods containing salicylates (including apples, cherries, grapes, aubergine, teas and coffee).

BOOST: Food intolerances can develop from eating too much of one thing. Vary your foods to avoid this.

TIP: If you suspect you have a food intolerance or an allergy have a look at the questionnaire at the back of this book (see page 169). If this indicates that you do, I would really recommend having a consultation with a qualified nutritional therapist.

GLUTEN

A link between endometriosis and gluten intolerance is being debated and is certainly far from scientifically proven as yet. Anecdotal evidence suggests that avoiding gluten, in wheat products in particular, can have a significantly positive impact on reducing or eliminating inflammation. I have seen this in a number of women in my clinic who have benefited from removing gluten from their diet, but it does take at least three months to make an optimum difference.

Remember that the protein gluten is not only in wheat; it is also in rye, barley and spelt. It is questionable whether oats also contain gluten but many people who cannot tolerate gluten feel better avoiding oats too. It is also used as a food additive in the form of a flavouring, stabilising or thickening agent, often as dextrin. Check your food labels if you aren't sure.

In the early 1970s wheat was genetically modified and a hormone was added to strengthen the crop. This new way of growing attracted fungal growth on the crop and in order to deal with this, yet another hormone was added.[13] It is this artificial cocktail that has been blamed for the rising link between endometriosis and wheat, although the mechanism of how it occurs does need more research. In addition to this, wheat contains a substance called phytic acid that can leach key minerals (such as zinc) needed for a healthy immune system from the body.

If you think you have a gluten intolerance it is worth getting a blood test. Ask your doctor to test for the following:

- IgG-gliadin
- IgA-gliadin
- tTG antibody
- Total IgA immunoglobulin levels
- Ferritin (checks for iron stores)
- C-Reactive Protein (CRP) (checks for inflammation in the bowels).

If you are gluten intolerant most of these test results will come up high and your iron levels will be low. See 'Boost' (page 64) for foods rich in iron.

BOOST: There are now plenty of gluten-free foods easily available – see the Useful Contacts section (page 165) for more direction. Delicious and nurturing gluten-free grain alternatives are brown rice, quinoa and rice noodles.

TIP: Remember that if you still choose to eat some wheat after reading this, restrict your consumption to wholewheat pasta and bread. Wholewheat does not include granary bread and brown bread. These are marketing terms and are, essentially, white, refined bread with extras thrown in. Spelt is the 'virgin' original form of wheat and so is also a nutritionally dense wholewheat option.

THE WRONG SORT OF DAIRY

Dairy gets an awful lot of bad press for intolerances and ill health. It is thought to stimulate the production of mucus and to trigger an immune reaction in those with a genetic disposition to atopic allergies such as asthma, eczema and inflammatory conditions such as psoriasis and hay fever or arthritis.

There are plenty of women who are genuinely affected by a dairy intolerance and although I am a staunch believer that we eat and drink far too much dairy in the western world, I do not believe these intolerances stem from overload as much as from poor quality. I am convinced that the detrimental effects are in fact not so much to do with the dear old cows but more to do with our handling of dairy products. That is, we pile chemicals into the food the (non-organic) cows eat to increase their production, and then homogenise and pasteurise milk to remove a great deal of its goodness. Sadly even organic milk that you can buy in supermarkets goes through

FACTS ON THE WHITE STUFF

WHAT DOES PASTEURISED MEAN? Pasteurisation is a technique developed by Louis Pasteur to kill micro-organisms by heating the milk for a short time and then cooling it for storage and transportation. This also extends the shelf life. The process destroys the vitamin C content of raw milk.

WHAT IS UHT? A newer process, known as ultrapasteurisation or ultra-high temperature treatment, which heats the milk to a higher temperature for a shorter amount of time. This allows the milk to be stored unrefrigerated for long periods.

WHAT IS HOMOGENISATION? Homogenisation is a treatment that prevents a cream layer from separating out of the milk. It is not a legal requirement, more of a cosmetic one. Homogenisation has no effect on shelf life. The milk is pumped at high pressures through very narrow tubes, breaking up the fat globules so that they can no longer rise to the top and develop a 'cream line'. I do not know about you, but as a kid I would get so excited about being the one to get the 'cream line'.

a process of homogenisation and pasteurisation. I do not believe this benefits our health in the way that we might like to think.

Proper, 'raw' milk from organic, well-nourished cows contains a fabulous cocktail of essential fats, protein, vitamins and minerals, as well as beneficial bacteria and lactase – the enzyme missing in individuals who are truly intolerant to dairy. Pasteurising and homogenising remove these; without them you cannot digest lactose and digestive disturbances and intolerance can begin. Raw milk therefore provides the 'full package' to be able to deal with intolerances and resultant allergies.

According to anecdotal evidence from both my own clinic and those of fellow health professionals, raw milk can help eczema, hay fever, allergies and asthma. In my house we have raw organic milk delivered to our door each morning and the entire family drinks it. Even my youngest child drinks it despite having had a bout of eczema in the past. His skin now retains the appearance of a beautiful baby's bottom all over. Raw organic milk has to carry the warning 'Caution: this milk could be bad for your health'. This is an interesting comment when we live in a world that is creating 'super bugs' because of our extreme hygiene.

In cases where my clients have self-diagnosed themselves to be 'dairy intolerant' I

BOOST: If you decide that dairy really is not for you, suitable alternatives are organic soya milk, rice or almond milk. Calcium is dense in nuts, chickpeas, tofu and dark green vegetables so you can ensure your calcium intake via these means instead. In order for the body to absorb calcium effectively it also needs a high magnesium content and these foods contain an ample supply of this mineral (it is not so high in cow's milk).

TIP: Try avoiding dairy for three months to see if your symptoms improve (your immune system is thought to have a memory of three months so a shorter trial may be inconclusive). After this you could try to reintroduce raw milk to see if the symptoms come back.

urge them to swap to raw milk before avoiding dairy completely, and to limit their intake. A healthy intake for anyone is around a half to a full mug of milk a day. By following the Nurture Diet you are likely to reduce dairy intake by default.

If you are pregnant the current health recommendations are to avoid dairy products that are unpasteurised. They are also not recommended for children under the age of five or the elderly. For anyone under medical supervision do check with your medical supervisor and ensure that the raw milk is produced at a reputable farm – see Further Help for more information (page 165).

FINAL WORD

The aim of the Nurture Diet is to remove negative foods and nourish your body with superior nutrient-rich foods, supplementing deficiency in vitamins and minerals to promote continual healing. Once the body is replenished with the nutritional building blocks it needs, it can work to reduce the inflammation and heal the existing damage caused by endometriosis. It is a long-term change; you could call it a lifestyle change rather than a diet. Here is a re-cap on the Nurture Diet:

DAILY:
- Eat a variety and plentiful amounts of fruit and vegetables.
- Eat complex carbohydrates – wholegrains such as brown rice, millet, rye and oats.
- Buy organic meat, dairy, fruit and vegetables where possible.
- Eat oily foods, including fish (3 times per week), nuts, seeds and oils.
- Avoid sugar, both on its own and hidden in foods.
- Drink 1.5 litres of filtered water per day.

AT LEAST THREE TIMES A WEEK:
- Eat your beans – phyto-estrogen-rich pulses such as lentils, chickpeas and soya beans.
- Have a 'red meat free' day – chose pulses, eggs, fish or poultry instead.
- Have an alcohol-free 24 hours.
- Have a caffeine-free day.

LIVING CONSCIOUSLY 4

Traditional Chinese medicine (TCM) is based on the concept of *yin* and *yang*; the shady side and the sunny side of the hill. *Yang* is considered to be the active form and *yin* the passive resting state. The Chinese believe health to be dependent on the balance between the two states. According to these principles if you lead a life that is too *yang*, always 'on the go' or persistently working, without giving yourself enough time to rest and relax (*yin*), your health can fall out of balance and conditions such as endometriosis can progress.

In this chapter we will look at the areas of your life that you can change to improve your experience of endometriosis. Previously you may not have been aware of the impact these factors may have on your health – I hope that the following indicates small changes that can make a real difference.

THE IMPORTANCE OF EXERCISE AND LIGHT

Get out for a blitz in the open air every day – in your lunch break, after work or with the kids. This is especially important if you work in an air-conditioned, strip-lit office.

Light itself is nourishment and a fabulous source of immune-supporting vitamin D. Vitamin D is necessary for the normal metabolism of calcium and phosphorus; both of these nutrients have important functions in the hormonal system.

Too much artificial lighting and too little natural light affects the entire body, including hormones and natural circadian rhythms. Production of the sleep hormone melatonin in the pineal gland is controlled by light and dark. When there is too little light, the body does not shut down the production of melatonin in the morning. This can lead to depression, listlessness and weight gain.

Exercise is important for general well-being, but even more so for those with endometriosis. It also encourages circulation to the pelvic area and moderates the overproduction of hormones. Getting the blood circulating encourages the optimum functioning of the bowels, which is important in eliminating waste products, including excess oestrogen. Exercise releases endorphins, which help us to feel happier, more alert and calmer. These brain chemicals improve low mood and anxiety, both of which can come about as a result of endometriosis. An exercise routine does not have to mean going to the gym three days a week or thrashing it out in an aerobics class. It can be getting off the bus a few stops earlier on your way to work, taking a stroll during your lunch break or signing up for a yoga course or swimming.

Yoga uses breathing techniques and postures to assist relaxation and healing. It encourages the 'free flow' of an internal energy called *prana* in Indian or 'Ayurvedic' medicine, or *chi* in Chinese medicine. It is thought that in conditions such as endometriosis this *prana* is not flowing freely and that the postures and breathing adopted during yoga can encourage it to circulate effectively again. Yoga supports blood circulation and the optimum flow of nutrients to all organs. Always use a qualified yoga teacher; to find an instructor local to you, contact the British Wheel of Yoga (see page 164).

If you are up for something more energetic, six months of aerobic activity (brisk walking four times a week for 30 minutes for example) has been shown to reverse the damage of 30 years of internal wear and tear. For every one per cent of added muscle mass, we can add 18 months to our lives. Regular exercising is paramount to good health.

I think it is crazy that the gym culture we have created is taking over as an alternative to exercising in the natural environment. The benefits of exercise come as a package: fresh air and a natural view, not an air-conditioned, soulless environment that breeds bacteria and dehydrates, whilst watching TV screens. That said, any activity in any form is better than doing nothing.

THINK, DRINK PURE

All drinking water should find its way through a filter within your home. Whether it's a water filter jug or a sophisticated plugged in system, *anything* is better than *nothing*. If you are using a water filter jug, do replace the filters regularly as these can become a breeding ground for bacteria.

However, investing in your health by spending the extra pennies on a sophisticated water filter system such as the 'reverse osmosis' system is undeniably worth it in my opinion. These filters remove the unwanted material, such as chlorine and xeno-oestrogens, but keep in the trace minerals, managing the job fantastically. Being an owner of one of these systems I can vouch for the superior quality of the water first-hand. The filter system forces the water under pressure through a semi-permeable membrane and allows you as much water as you want. Very often the pressure flow is not that far off a 'normal' tap. They are inexpensive to run but do take up space under your sink. I think you will find that after years of buying new filters for standard water systems the initial financial outlay for a reverse osmosis system will be no more expensive.

Or you could live off glass-bottled water. As mentioned before, plastic bottles increase the body's toxic load of xeno-oestrogens because the plastic compounds can leach into the water content, further contributing to oestrogen dominance in women with endometriosis.

A healthy water intake (1.5 litres a day) encourages the elimination of daily external and internal toxins; it maximises energy, revitalises the appearance of skin and balances mineral levels. The World Health Organization has gone as far as to say that 80 per cent of the world's illnesses would be eliminated if we all drank pure water. Usually we need around 1–1.5 litres per day but as you begin to drink water regularly you will find your body regulating your needs. The need is also flexible according to the weather, how much exercise you take and how many dehydrating drinks or foods (salty foods, caffeine, alcohol) you have consumed that day. If you exercise, ensure you drink a few glasses more to compensate. Coffee, tea, sugar, air travel or air-conditioned offices are all dehydrating too so add in extra for these. Do not wait for your body to feel thirsty, by this stage you are already dehydrated. Dehydration can also be disguised as hunger or a craving for salty food, so check it is not a glass of water you need rather than a packet of crisps! Herbal teas, fruit and veg also have a high water content and count towards your water intake. My top tip is to buy a 1.5 litre glass bottle of water to begin with and aim to finish it by the end of the day – not just before you go to bed or you will be up in the night. Keep it with you on your desk, in the car, nearby when you are doing your daily activities. The next day either buy a new one or fill up a glass bottle from your own water filter system and continue. Drink between meals throughout the day, avoiding the common mistake of only remembering to drink with meals. This tends to result in gulping a glass of water and will only help to flush the nutrients through the digestive system too quickly, making them hard to absorb.

BALANCED WEIGHT, BALANCED HORMONES

As discussed in the previous chapter, fat cells contain the oestrogen-promoting enzyme aromatase. Therefore the more fat cells you have the more oestrogen is produced. Maintaining a healthy weight is key in balancing your hormones and thereby tackling endometriosis naturally. Following the Nurture Diet, as well as exercising, can vastly help to bring your weight into balance. Note that being underweight can also be detrimental to health and hormone balance, so here I am talking about a medically healthy weight, not the weight you may see promoted on catwalks. Although many in the medical field determine your healthy weight by your body mass index (BMI), this measurement does not take into consideration your fat or lean body mass. I feel it is this ratio between fat percentage and lean body mass that is the most important. As I have already stressed, fat, or adipose tissue, can negatively affect oestrogen levels – not having enough fat on your body or having too much. You can be a low weight but have a high body fat count or vice versa. If you are in the market for buying new scales I would really recommend some body fat scales as these will tell you how much of your weight is made up of fat. Healthy body fat ratio should be between 21–30 per cent in a woman aged 25–40 years old.

ARE YOU STRESSED?

Sometimes you have to wait for your soul to catch up with your body.

Chinese proverb

One of the greatest problems with modern life is the emotional and mental toxicity it can bring. We can spend so much time outside ourselves and so little time being present and able to listen to our own bodies and our intuition. Our spirit and our physical body can become two separate entities. This is not a healthy state to be in. Taking time to relax and come 'back together' is extremely important for total health.

Modern society exposes us to many stressful experiences. As individuals we may not be aware of these 'minor' stresses but cumulatively, over time, they can exhaust health. Examples include high noise levels; lack of free time; excessive exercise; no opportunity to process emotions; high demands on performance, which can be self-inflicted or placed on you by colleagues or family at work and at home; being on the receiving end of, or regularly witnessing, unpleasant behaviour. Some of these stress factors can be especially common in cities and urban areas. They wear down the health of the spirit, which in turn wears down the physical elements of our being.

When we are stressed the adrenal glands prompt the release of glucose and stress hormones into the bloodstream, triggering what we know as the 'fight or flight' response. In caveman days this was a useful response to a sabre-toothed tiger or a woolly mammoth and we would respond by running or fighting, either of which used up the sudden release of glucose and hormones. Once the threatening event had passed, our system would more or less be neutralised by the exact science of supply and demand. Today our source of stress is not a ferocious wild animal but our children/work/late bus/finances/partner, none of which requires physical fighting or running away – as much as at times we may want to. This means that the glucose and hormones released are not used but continue to circulate in the bloodstream making our symptoms worse. Additionally, our bodies can crave sugar-laden food or a stimulant.

If this happens on a continual basis, which it does for so many of us, the adrenal glands become increasingly overworked and undernourished, causing chaos in the production and regulation of our hormones. By the time the adrenals are exhausted we can become more prone to anger, illness, irritability, excessive sweating and depression. The hormone released to cope with this is cortisol. Cortisol competes with and lowers progesterone production and therefore contributes to a dominance of oestrogen. Stress management, therefore, is essential to any woman with endometriosis.

Meditation, yoga, moderate exercise and massage are all tried-and-tested, valid approaches to reducing stress. My tip would be to choose the right way to unwind that suits *you*, not your neighbour or colleague at work, but *you*. Stick to it and be disciplined in making sure you find time for it in your schedule; it is so important to find time to breathe.

GETTING ENOUGH SLEEP

Sleep is a time of cellular repair. Any damage done during the day gets a chance to be repaired and balance restored. Too little sleep makes it much harder to handle stresses, both mental and environmental. Tiredness also makes us more prone to choosing unhealthy foods such as refined carbohydrates, sugar-laden foods or caffeine. This raises the level of stress hormones and can heighten hormonal imbalance. Some women find that this initiates a vicious cycle as they are disturbed by the symptoms of hormone imbalance, such as night sweats or waking up at three or four a.m. as the detoxification systems work even harder.

Magnetic imbalances (see page 82) affect our sleep cycle making it difficult to get the deep sleep we need to be truly rested. A good tip is either to avoid electrical appliances in the bedroom or to unplug them at night. Common culprits are charging your mobile phone by your bedside, digital alarm clocks or electric blankets.

If you are finding it difficult to wake up, lack energy during the day and rely on caffeine to get you through and/or yawn a lot, you are not getting enough sleep. Better quality sleep is something that can be achieved through following a cleansing diet.

Whether it is going to sleep in the first place or staying asleep that is the problem, mental anxiety and emotional concerns can also interfere with a solid night's sleep. Remove the tangible and intangible clutter as much as you can before going to bed. Clear your room of mess, have a relaxing bath with sedative essential oils such as lavender or neroli, and even dab a little on your pillow. Get snuggly – holding a hot water bottle for warmth can be soporific. Adopt the habit of going to bed at a regular time. Don't eat too late (at least 3 hours before retiring). Keep fresh air circulating through the bedroom; oxygen enables the sleep centre to do its thing better. Relaxation techniques such as meditation or visualisation can help the mind to switch off. If anxiety is at the root of the insomnia, herbal medicine has some effective natural remedies such as passiflora, camomile, valerian or rhodiola. These herbs can be taken as a tincture remedy put together by a herbalist or taken as a tablet or tea before bed. They can take a week or so to start working effectively and so it is important to give them this time at least. It is also important to see them as 'part of the picture'. By this I mean you also need to look at reducing the stress factors that are causing you anxiety in the first place.

HOW IS YOUR ENVIRONMENTAL STRESS? ELECTROMAGNETIC RADIATION AND GEOPATHIC STRESS

The body emits a broad spectrum of electromagnetic radiation and disruption to this can disturb sleep and the hormone cycle. Such disruptions include electromagnetic radiation from electric blankets, sunbeds, mobile phones and their masts, walk-about home phones and baby monitors. These areas have received a lot of interest as being potential contributors to cancer[1] – the World Health Organization (WHO) has classified electromagnetic radiation from mobile phones as a possible carcinogen. The chairman of the working group for this WHO research stated: 'the evidence, while still accumulating, is strong enough to support a conclusion and the 2B classification (probably carcinogenic to humans). The conclusion means that there could be some risk, and therefore we need to keep a close watch for a link between cell phones and cancer risk . . . Given the potential consequences for public health of this classification and findings . . .it is important to take pragmatic measures to reduce exposure such as hands-free devices or texting.' The strongest link (40 per cent increase in risk) is in heavy users, defined as 30 minutes of use daily for ten years. As many use mobile phones as their main form of communication a significant amount of people will fall into this category. Although research needs to confirm these findings, studies so far have also demonstrated that mobile phones may have a marked negative effect on fertility rates.[2]

Research has shown that electromagnetic fields from mobile phones affect memory and the immune system. A study of specific immune cells known as leukotrienes showed that only one third of the cells survived after three hours of exposure to a mobile phone.[3] In her book *The Self-Healing Human*, the immunologist Susanna Ehdin discussed the concept of the 'female immune system' and that female sex hormones, including oestrogen and progesterone, play a major role in regulating the female immune system and vice versa. The female reproductive system and immune systems are so intimately linked that fluctuations in the sex hormones (such as excess levels of oestrogen) can affect the immune system. This tallies with observational studies that show women can have reduced immunity during menstruation, pregnancy and menopause, only to regain their immune strength as soon as any of these is over. If the sex hormone levels are continually out of sync, as is the case with endometriosis sufferers, it leaves the women more prone to infection.

Women who spend more than 20 hours a week in front of visual display unit (VDU) screens may have an increased chance of miscarriage and research has shown that men who are very active users of mobile phones or have them on standby throughout the day have significantly lower sperm concentration.[4] These findings are noteworthy but require further research to confirm the link. Commonplace items such as digital alarm clocks, TVs, DVD players, laptops or power sockets near your bed may also increase your exposure to this electromagnetic radiation. Try turning them off when you don't need them, or even better removing them and replacing them with battery operated alternatives.

Traditional Chinese medicine (TCM) reinforces the idea that electromagnetic radiation can affect our *qi* (life energy). According to Pythagoras, this is the vital energy that leads to the body's healing.[5] Pythagoras and other ancient Greek philosophers believed that because mathematical concepts were more 'practical' (easier to regulate and classify) than physical ones, they had greater actuality.

TCM, and its associated fields such as acupuncture, base their science on this theory of numeracy or 'mystical numerical associations', being the basis of locating acupuncture points.[6]

BE CONSCIOUS OF WHAT YOU PUT IN AND ON YOUR BODY

Bleached tampons and sanitary towels are a controversial area in the endometriosis debate. Tampons such as those produced by major manufacturers use bleached paper products and now, commonly, bleached card or plastic applicators. This bleaching process used to produce dioxins as a by-product of the manufacturing process of sanitary towels, tampons, loo paper and nappies.[7] As I have already mentioned in previous chapters, dioxins been shown to have an adverse affect the immune and reproductive system.[8,9] Nowadays tampon manufacturers use a different bleaching method – chlorine dioxide instead of chlorine bleach – although a study conducted by the FDA Office of Women's Health in 2005 found detectable levels of dioxin still present in seven tampons brands. This raises concerns over the release of dioxins into the atmosphere and water as part of the incineration or disposal of this domestic waste. Ordinarily the vagina is an oxygen-free environment, preventing the growth of bacteria. However, using tampons can disrupt this as oxygen can become trapped in the fibres, increasing the possibility of toxin and bacterial overgrowth. This also increases the risk of these toxins and bacteria entering the bloodstream. Using 100% organic cotton sanitary products, although still vulnerable to trace amounts of dioxins, greatly minimises the vagina's exposure to harmful chemicals and I and other health experts urge you to use these in place of larger non-organic cotton brands.[10] I know that using sanitary towels in the day is not a first choice for many women but where possible try to minimise your use of tampons (100% organic cotton or not), saving their use for occasions such as swimming or when on holiday (Natracare are a good brand, see page 166). Where you cannot avoid using tampons, ensure you change them after a maximum of 3 hours. These products are not always as effective at absorbing the blood flow so you may feel you have to change them more regularly anyway.

It has been suggested that a woman may use as many as 11,000 tampons in her lifetime, and this represents a worrying level of dioxin exposure to a very delicate area of the female body. With the younger onset of menstruation could this explain the increasing incidence of endometriosis in young women?

Some health experts argue that tampons encourage 'retrograde' flow by pushing the blood back into the system rather than removing it and I happen to agree with this too.[11]

Reducing our toxic load can be simple; it just needs consciousness. Changes to diet and household choices can reduce exposure to a remarkable degree and ease the pressure on the body. It is important to pay close attention to your choice of household chemicals and toiletries.

Anti-perspirant deodorants often contain aluminium. Aluminium is a metal that easily attaches itself to DNA within cells and stays there. As it is the nearest fatty tissue to the armpit, the breast is particularly vulnerable to the possible harmful effects. Although applying an anti-perspirant might feel like a necessity when wearing a new top in summer, sweating is another way of eliminating toxins; therefore preventing the sweating blocks toxin removal. Ironically if your toxin load is great, sweating can increase and you may be more inclined to reach for the 24-hour anti-perspirant, and so the cycle continues. Balancing your hormonal status through a cleansing diet should address any excess sweating and hopefully remove the need to use anti-perspirants. Deodorants, on the other hand, mask the smell of sweat rather than blocking the excretory pores and are therefore preferable. An easily available brand is Bionsen in either a pump spray or roll-on.

Soaps wash away natural fatty acids, beneficial bacteria and enzymes found in the skin, disrupt the natural pH level and interfere with the skin's protective role. Shampoos containing natural glycerine are gentler on the scalp and can make us less vulnerable to psoriasis or dandruff. Skin lotions and lip balms mostly contain paraffin or mineral oils made from crude oil that paradoxically have a drying effect on the skin and lips. They also put a greater strain on the liver and immune system. If the skin's protective barrier is breached continually, the immune system must deal with the invaders that have seeped in, giving it much more work. Many cosmetics also contain parabens (that mimic the effects of oestrogen in the body and have been named as a contributing factor in breast cancer) and it is estimated that women are exposed to 50mg of parabens daily from their cosmetics and personal care products alone. Not good news for women with any type of hormone disruption, including endometriosis.

So what can you do? It is a good idea to examine your skincare and hygiene products and switch to those without chemical foaming agents (sodium laurel sulphate), acrylamides, mineral oils and parabens (these usually have a prefix before paraben such as methylparaben). Choosing organic skincare products and make up wherever possible will limit your exposure to these greatly. Make it a rule not to buy a product with an ingredient that you don't recognise or cannot pronounce as these are often toxic culprits! See Appendix 2 for organic and toxin-free skincare products as well as further reading on this subject.

For household cleaning products, you can buy alternative products that don't contain harmful ingredients *or* get the vinegar and baking soda out and start making your own – economical and good for you. See Appendix 6 (page 174) for more information on what to look out for.

Environmental toxins are hard to avoid if you live a busy modern life, but they are not impossible to reduce. Being conscious about the toiletries and household products that you buy will soon become a habit and you will find that your choices will naturally be 'cleaner'.

LOOKING AFTER YOUR EMOTIONAL WELL-BEING

Sometimes we can become trapped in our emotions. Our feelings are the path to ourselves and to healing and if we try to anaesthetise these unhealed emotions, we can anaesthetise our essence and our health.

Suzannah Ehdin

The rapidly growing science of psycho-neuro-immunology (PNI) has shown that our state of mind directly affects the functioning of all tissues in the body. High levels of prolonged physical stress and emotional distress can flatten the immune system.

The reasons we overeat, smoke, drink excessively or indulge in other self-destructive habits are often because we are anxious, lonely, lost, bored, angry or depressed. Unless we understand and process these emotions, our mental and physical health can take a battering. Nurturing your self-care and self-esteem provides a sustainable basis for health and recovery.

The view of the human body in western medicine is based on anatomical studies, while more eastern views (such as Ayurvedic or Traditional Chinese Medicine) are based on life energy – qi and prana, translated as breathing and life. Pythagoras identified this need for life's energy over 2,500 years ago and believed it was this that was at the very core of healing from disease. According to these more holistic views on well-being there are three stages of health: the physical, the emotional and life's energy itself (soul or 'spirit'). These energy levels interact with one another and if they are not in harmony we lose energy and physical disease occurs.[12] In other words, it is difficult for your body to be healthy if your mind and soul are not.

Like other women with endometriosis, you may have had a long, emotionally draining journey to get a diagnosis. In the process you may not have been listened to by those professionals from whom you sought advice. Your intuition that something was wrong may not have been valued.

After years of battling with your own health you can find yourself entrenched in negative memories of health, hostage to your own physical body.

You cannot get away from the fact that you will be spending the rest of your life with yourself. This can be an uphill struggle if you spend it criticising yourself and feeling victimised. Self-acceptance can take the struggle out of life so that you can concentrate on true healing. Do not mistake this as complacency. What I am referring to is about accepting, respecting and improving your whole self. The drive for self-improvement is healthy when it comes from a place of love and respect rather than a feeling of inadequacy.

Inviting change is the first step to supporting healing. Focus on what it is that you want – less pain, improved energy – and how it is holding you back from life. Visualise what that would look and feel like. Colour yourself in it. Engage with the emotion that comes with it – do you feel lighter, happier? How would it impact on your life – would you be able to engage in more social occasions? Would you be able to enjoy sex more? Do it, make it happen. By acting in a way you would prefer to be you are sending a message to your unconscious that you want to feel well.

This does not take away the reality of the physical but it might go a long way in improving your experience of endometriosis.

There is an undeniable physiological link between emotional health and the health of the digestive system. The gut has over 100 million neurons and neural tissue, second only to the brain, and an overactive inflammatory response is also now thought to induce feelings of depression.[13,14,15] As the digestive system often needs support in endometriosis and inflammation is notably heightened, these may contribute to the development of associated depression.

Studies also suggest that an imbalance in oestrogen and progesterone levels negatively affect our endorphin production (those clever chemicals that make us feel good).[16] Our emotions can affect our physical defences too and repressed emotions may also weaken the immune system.[17] Addressing your thoughts and emotions can simultaneously affect the strength of your immune system and the biochemistry within your brain.

Failing to honour yourself can create emotional disharmony that can take its toll on the body. For some, finding harmony may require the help of a therapist, meditation or a spiritual practice. Finding what you need in order to achieve this goal may be a process of elimination, but it could be the vital piece the jigsaw of health that is currently missing.

MANAGING YOUR ENDOMETRIOSIS WITH SUPPLEMENTS
Supplements receive a mixed press and there is a lot of confusion amongst the public about whether or not we should take supplements, let alone which ones.

Optimum, therapeutic levels of nutrients are key in taking control of your endometriosis. Sadly, a diet that provides us with the complete spectrum of nutrients our body requires is harder to achieve than in times gone by. Mass production farming techniques mean that much of the soil in which food is grown is depleted of its mineral content, which means we are not receiving our ideal nutrient supply from food. This said, supplements are not a health insurance whereby we can pop a couple of pills and eat and drink a high calorie, low nutrient diet. We must do everything we can to reach our nutrient requirements through food with supplements as a 'top up'.

With pre-existing conditions the body may need more than a gentle helping hand. If your health problem has been underlying for some time, as is commonly the case with endometriosis, the body's natural healing processes can become worn down and less able to manage your condition on their own. It is at this point that your body will begin to show visible signs that it is not faring well. With endometriosis the body needs the extra support that supplements can give. Research shows that taking the right nutrients in food supplements can reduce the symptoms of endometriosis significantly (98 per cent of the women in one study experienced improvements).[18]

When I began to write this book I had the simple intention of putting what I know down on paper. Through my research, however, I came to the conclusion that there was nothing out there specifically for women with endometriosis that I felt able to recommend. For example, many of the formulas to support a cleansing programme contained alfalfa; high doses of this plant are best avoided in hormone-related conditions. My work has involved formulating health products for other health companies in the past and I have now formulated a small range of premium food supplements specifically for women with endometriosis and conditions characterised by oestrogen dominance. They include the following nutrients that have been shown to be especially effective in the management of endometriosis. For more information on these products please refer to Useful Contacts (page 162). I truly believe in these products; I take them myself and *know* that they have supported my return to full health. Regardless of which brand you go for, do make sure they contain these ingredients and remember that you do get what you pay for, spending a little extra on quality products can make a significant difference to the outcome. Not all nutrient forms are equal; there are a number of different forms that you can buy. For example the minerals zinc and magnesium are most bioavailable in the citrate and ascorbate forms. This means that your body can use them more efficiently and as a result you do end up getting greater benefits for your money. Other forms may pass through your body without being absorbed so that in fact, although cheaper to buy initially, they end up being more expensive in terms of value for money. You need to read the labels carefully.

If you are on any kind of medication, have high blood pressure or diabetes, check with your medical consultant or GP before commencing.

- **Methionine** supports the detoxification process of the liver, especially in the breakdown of excess oestrogen.
- **The B vitamin group** is key in any holistic approach to endometriosis. Choline and B12 are lipotropic factors that hasten the removal or decrease the deposition of fat and bile in the liver therefore helping liver function and the removal of toxins. B6 is vital in the breakdown and regulation of oestrogen as well as significantly reducing the intensity and duration of period pains.[19] The B vitamin family is also vital in the conversion of the important fatty acid GLA. GLA supports the production of anti-inflammatory mediators that can reduce the pain-associated inflammation in endometriosis and relax the muscles. The recommended dose is 100mg B complex per day.
- **Magnesium**, known as nature's tranquiliser, acts as a muscle relaxant and has been shown to have a beneficial effect on painful periods and lower back pain.[20,21,22] The recommended dose is 300mg per day.
- **Vitamin E** levels were found to be significantly lower in endometriosis sufferers according to recent research.[23,24] This could be the result of an increased oxidation process that occurs naturally in cases of inflammation. Vitamin E supplementation of 200iu taken twice a day has also been shown to relieve menstrual cramps in 70 per cent of women within two menstrual cycles.[25,26]

- **Vitamin C** levels are lower in sufferers of endometriosis and supplementation with this vitamin for six months has been shown to reduce oxidative stress significantly, thereby allowing healing.[27,28] Vitamin C supplements containing bioflavanoids are helpful with pain occurring around the time of your period as they help the muscle to relax and reduce inflammation.[29] The recommended dose is 500mg twice a day.

- **Zinc** works as an antioxidant by protecting the body's cells from free radical damage, and is also necessary for immune function. If zinc levels are low, the immune system will not function optimally because it needs zinc to fight off viruses and bacteria. The recommended dose is 15mg per day.

- **Pycnogenol** is a therapeutic alternative to GnRHa in the treatment of endometriosis and has been shown to have a marked effect on pain management and inflammation.[30] The recommended dose is 30mg twice a day.

- **Omega 3 essential fatty acids** are essential for healthy hormonal function and keeping inflammation in check. They are needed by every cell in the body. In a study conducted on women following a diet low in caffeine, sugar and dairy and supplementing their diet with fish oils the results demonstrated a significant reduction in pain in the pelvic area associated with endometriosis.[31] Oily fish is a great source of omega 3 but dietary intakes of these fats from food sources have declined in the past decade and consumption is now too low to meet recommendations for long-chain omega-3 fatty acids.[32] On top of this there is concern over the heavy metals and other toxins found in the seas in which they are fished. Quality fish oil supplements providing a minimum of 1000mg are a good way of boosting intake of omega 3 whilst being highly distilled to remove toxins. Krill oil is receiving a lot of positive reports on its delivery of omega 3 fatty acids and its anti-inflammatory benefits. If you are vegetarian I would recommend 1000mg of linseed (flaxseed) oil. Linseeds also contain lignans, which block oestrogen receptors in the cell and reduce the symptoms of oestrogen dominance in conditions like endometriosis.

- **Probiotics** If you feel your digestive system needs a bit of extra support then take a probiotic supplement. Probiotic bacteria can help to create a healthy intestinal environment, boosting immunity and promoting optimum digestion. Select a probiotic formula that contains at least two billion colony-forming units (CFUs) of acidophilus per dose.

With all the doses recommended take into consideration the levels of these nutrients in any other supplements you are taking, such as a multivitamin. The best piece of advice that I can give you is to make a concerted effort to stick to your supplement programme every day. It will not work as well if you dip in and out as and when you remember. Sit them in front of you on your desk at work or in a visible place at home – but out of the light and not above room temperature to avoid them being damaged. I put mine next to the sink taps so I cannot avoid seeing them.

HERBAL MEDICINE FOR ENDOMETRIOSIS

Experimental evidence is accumulating to suggest that medicinal botanicals have anti-inflammatory and pain-alleviating properties and hold promise for the treatment of endometriosis.[33] Herbs and nutrition have a wonderfully synergistic relationship. Taking herbs alongside a nurturing lifestyle can work both to support the diet in normalising hormone levels as well as being excellent for helping you to cope with the worst symptoms.[34] They also have a wonderful complementary effect alongside food supplements and are perfectly safe to take at the correct dosage and in combination. Clinical evidence has shown that herbal medicine has a regulatory effect on the circulatory, immune and hormonal systems.

The European Directive on Traditional Herbal Medicinal Products requires that all over-the-counter herbal medicinal products that are not fully licensed as medicines must have authorisation to be marketed within the EU. In order to obtain this authorisation a company needs to demonstrate that the herbal medicine has been in use within the EU for at least 30 years, or for 15 years within the EU and 30 years outside the EU. This legislation serves to regulate the quality and safety as well as the health claims of herbs for the sake of the public that use them. It may however limit our access to some traditional herbal medicines, which were in common use more than 30 years ago, but have since fallen into disuse. Sadly, it costs a lot of money for companies to 'license' their products to gain authorisation and therefore this directive has seen the closure of many brilliant but small herbal suppliers. The dosage at which these products can be marketed has also been capped, so that many therapeutic western herbs at effective doses are only available through a herbal practitioner. A number of the purely herbal products (i.e. only herbs in the product) sold 'off the shelf' from health food stores and supermarkets are not of optimum strength.

For the following information on herbal medicine I enlisted the wisdom of Michael McIntyre, the pioneering herbal practitioner, who has provided information and, where possible, therapeutic doses for endometriosis. I really would recommend a consultation with a herbal practitioner for an optimum formulation bespoke for you (see Useful Contacts, page 163).

WESTERN HERBS
For regulating oestrogen and progesterone levels and balance
- **Agnus-castus** otherwise known as chaste tree or vitex, agnus castus is an excellent herb for female hormone problems. It restores balance by reducing or raising hormone levels where appropriate by stimulating and normalising the function of the pituitary gland.[35] Usual dose is 1–5ml of tincture (1:2 extract) daily for long-term therapy. Higher doses may be used for short-term treatment of acute conditions but this is probably best done following professional advice.
- **Wild yam** (*Dioscorea villosa*) is used traditionally to redress progesterone insufficiency.[36] It is often thought to work because it blocks strong oestrogens, but its less well-known anti-inflammatory and anti-spasmodic effects may well be why it helps.[37,38] Dosage is variable and requires a consultation.

For pain management
- **Cramp bark** (*Viburnum opulus*), as the English name suggests, works as an anti-spasmodic and muscle relaxant. Dose is 5ml of tincture in water every four hours to relieve acute pain.
- **Turmeric** (*Curcuma longa*) The active ingredient in this wonderful spice is showing great promise in treating endometriosis due to its potent ability to reduce inflammation as well as its use as an antioxidant for repairing damage from endometrial adhesions and scar tissue.[39] The recommended dose is 400–

600mg of turmeric powder (standardised to curcumin content) three times per day. Use as much as you can in your cooking too.

*   **Dong gui** (*Angelica sinensis*) is used for heavy and painful periods and anaemia. It is given to invigorate the blood flow so may work to 'move' stagnant blood according to Traditional Chinese Medicine. It has been shown to engage with oestrogen receptors thereby reducing the amount of oestrogen used by the body when there is excess.[40] The recommended dose is 4ml tincture (1:5) in water three times per day.
*   **Yarrow** (*Achillea millefolium*) is a less researched herb used for menstrual irregularities and cramps.[41] It is anti-inflammatory and may have a use for endometriosis sufferers at the recommended dose of 2–4 ml tincture (1:5) in water three times per day.

To strengthen the immune system

*   **Echinacea** species include *E. purpurea, E. angustifolia* and *E. pallida*. Most people have heard of Echinacea, I am sure, because it receives a lot of press for its immune-supporting properties.[42] As the immune system is weakened in women with endometriosis this is a popular and effective herb. Dosage is 5ml tincture (1:5) three times daily in water. (No rest period is needed if trying to control symptoms: this is advice for warding off colds.)
*   **Elderberry** (*Sambucus negra*) is a lesser-known western herb but is by no means inferior in its ability to support the immune system. I think it is fantastic; a wolf in sheep's clothing – gentle on the system but powerful in its effects. Increasingly research is showing that this herb has an ability to modulate the immune system, calming and strengthening it and thereby offering anti-inflammatory effects. Elderberry extract can also strengthen the body's defences against viral and bacterial infections, both of which women with endometriosis may be more prone to.[43,44] Dosage is 5ml of extract four times daily.

For supporting emotional and mental well-being

*   **St John's Wort** (*Hypericum perforatum*) is well known for its mood stabilising effects and can be a suitable alternative to prescription antidepressants without the side effects. Research suggests that St John's Wort can lift mood within three

weeks of starting the course and can be as effective as the selective serotonin reuptake inhibitor (SSRI) fluoxetine (Prozac) in improving mood, decreasing anxiety and reducing insomnia related to depression.[45,46] Although natural remedies can work wonders in the area of depression, for symptoms other than mild depression/low mood I highly recommend that you discuss these options with your GP before embarking on any course of treatment. The recommended dose for endometriosis is 300mg three times per day of a standardised extract providing at least 0.3 per cent of hypericin, best taken after food. St John's Wort must not be taken with antidepressants or several other prescription drugs such as the anticoagulant warfarin, cholesterol-lowering medication such as simvastatin or protease inhibitors and may even make the contraceptive pill ineffective. Consult your doctor before taking with any other medication. There is some good evidence that the overall effect of St John's Wort is to increase the level of the 'feel good' brain chemicals serotonin, noradrenaline and dopamine, which can have a dramatic effect upon depression and overall well-being.

• **Roseroot** (*Rhodiola rosea*) is up there with my favourite herbs – and this is saying something as herbs rock for endometriosis! It is used for increasing energy, stamina, strength and mental capacity, and to help the body adapt to and resist physical, chemical and environmental stress. It is also used for improving athletic performance, sexual function, depression, anxiety – sounding good for the management of endometriosis isn't it? Roseroot is also used for preventing colds and flu; treating cancer, ageing, liver damage; strengthening the nervous system and enhancing immunity. For depression it has been shown to reduce mild-to-moderate symptoms after six weeks of treatment.[47] It has also been shown to reduce mental fatigue, reduce anxiety and improve mental performance such as memory.[48,49] Dosage for endometriosis is 340mg twice daily.

TRADITIONAL CHINESE MEDICINE

Scientific research is increasingly showing how effective Traditional Chinese Medicine (TCM) can be for the treatment of conditions that affect the female endocrine system. TCM convention emphasises the importance of a healthy and balanced blood flow in women for good reproductive health. A recent study [50,51] is the first English-language systematic review [52] of Chinese Herbal Medicine (CHM;

one string of the TCM bow) for the treatment of endometriosis. The researchers analysed, in particular, two trials of 158 women in total. In one clinical trial, therapy with Chinese herbs provided a reduction of symptoms that was comparable to the relief provided by the hormone medication Gestrinone. And the herbs, unlike the drug, caused few side effects. In the second trial, CHM was even more successful in treating endometriosis than the hormonal drug Danazol. Again, the Chinese herbs produced fewer side effects than the western medication.

I have worked with experts in TCM who say that endometriosis is a symptom of a state known as 'blood stagnation'. Blood stagnation can be remedied with a multi-disciplinary approach, using herbal medicine, acupuncture and dietary changes, most of which we have discussed already.

ACUPUNCTURE

Acupuncture operates on the belief that the body is comprised of many different pathways or 'meridians'. Along these acupuncture meridians runs an energy force known as *qi*. If *qi* becomes blocked or stagnates anywhere along a pathway, it will cause the body to become imbalanced and produce physical symptoms, such as pain or illness. By stimulating the energy through various acupuncture points found along the meridians, *qi* can flow freely again, helping the body regain its balance. This is undertaken by inserting fine, sterile needles along specific pathways and at certain points according to the symptoms.

Acupuncture has been widely acknowledged in the natural health and medical community for its benefits in treating endometriosis by promoting the body's healing responses, stimulating the flow of energy through the body and helping to restore balance. Improved uterine blood flow also has important implications for women undergoing in-vitro fertilisation (IVF). It is also proven to encourage the body to produce endorphins to reduce pain (and, as I have seen in many women in my clinic, produces wonderful results).[53, 54]

I recently read about a couple of interesting studies that suggest 'medical management of pain in women with endometriosis is currently inadequate for many. Possibly acupuncture . . . may be used as an adjunct'.[55] In a study published in the December 2002 issue of the *Journal of Traditional Chinese Medicine* researchers selected 67 women diagnosed with dysmenorrhoea (painful periods) due to endometriosis. It was reported that 81 per cent of those women who had acupuncture had less painful periods after receiving the acupuncture treatments.[56]

BLOOD STAGNATION TEA: A lovely tea recipe by a colleague and friend of mine, Emma Cannon: Simmer equal parts of cinnamon, ginger and tangerine peel in water until you have reduced the tea by a third, then drink. Delicious! Feel the blood circulate . . .

FINAL WORD
The strength of a nurturing approach to health depends on your own engagement with the healing process. You can take control of your potential health and happiness by making small but powerful changes to the way you live. Just becoming conscious is the start of the process. An improved experience of endometriosis depends on a total body approach, and addressing your lifestyle and emotions play a pivotal role.

A recap on how you can live consciously:

Everyday:
- Take a vitamin and mineral supplement tailored to support hormone balance and antioxidant formula (containing the nutrients listed). See Useful Contacts.
- Get outside for some fresh air and light. Getting out for a walk or exercise such as yoga first thing in the morning is great for kickstarting the circulation and flow of nutrients around the body. It also helps to maintain a healthy weight.
- Drink plenty (1.5 litres) of filtered water a day. Look into installing a water filter where you live.
- Deep breathe. This helps you to relax and de-stress as well as encouraging oxygen to circulate, improving energy and healing.

◆ Get your shut-eye. Sleep gives the body the opportunity to regenerate and repair wear and tear from the day. If it is not given this space, damage can accumulate and conditions such as hormonal imbalance can occur.

What else can you do?

◆ Check your geopathic stress. Remove wi-fi systems, phones and digital alarm clocks from your bedroom and use hands-free kits for mobile telephones to reduce your exposure to electromagnetic fields.

◆ Be conscious of what you put in and on your body. Choose organic skincare products without ingredients such as parabens, mineral oils, acrylamides and unbleached sanitary products.

◆ Chose 'natural' cleaning products for your home, to reduce the number of potentially xeno-estrogenic chemicals in your house.

◆ Remove plastic wrapping from bought foods before putting them away to store in a cupboard or fridge.

◆ Chose aluminium-free deodorants. These are available from good health food shops and some supermarkets. Aluminium will be listed in the ingredients list if present so read the label before buying.

◆ Look after your emotional well-being. Take the time to look after yourself and your emotions; you can easily become worn down by stress and leave yourself vulnerable to further physical ill health.

◆ Consider consulting an acupuncturist or herbal practitioner for complementary treatments to your diet or to address hormonal balance or pain.

GETTING GOING 5

So you have read the book up to this point, and I hope have realised the need to make a change and take care of yourself. You may feel that, as much as you would like to make these changes, you simply haven't got the time. Perhaps this it true, perhaps you do have a very busy job, or a house full of demanding children or a partner that will only eat meat and two veg, but it is not an excuse. You can find the time, and believe me if you do so, the changes will find you the energy. By taking care of yourself, you do, in turn, take care of others. This might be the ideal moment to take stock and assess whether your priorities are where they should be for your long-term health.

This chapter is about summarising the dietary and lifestyle changes addressed so far and putting them into an action plan to get you going.

I do understand that old habits die hard. That is a psychological fact. But with commitment they do, eventually, keel over. There is no point pretending that change is easy – it isn't. It will take a while before the new lifestyle starts to feel natural and comfortable but as you begin to feel the benefits you may wonder why you never did it before.

Identify the triggers that trip you up. Do you get a 'blood sugar dip' after lunch? Do you arrive home starving to an empty fridge? Are you keeping yourself hydrated? Remember thirst can be mistaken for hunger. Be organised by planning ahead and shopping online so the kitchen is well stocked with the right foods.

Be gentle on yourself. There may well be periods where you slip into old habits. This does not mean all is lost, and faltering is sometimes part of your journey to healthy eating. When or if you do fall off track, don't beat yourself up. Guilt and chastisement are self-defeating. With the knowledge you now have you can pick yourself up and take one day at a time, paving your way to fixing nurturing habits. Allow three months for the changes to get to work properly on your health.

The advice in this chapter and throughout the book does not mean that you can never have a late night, drink unfiltered water or eat non-organic carrots ever again. Getting it right 80 per cent of the time can be enough.

PUTTING IT INTO ACTION

Take time to establish these new habits. Spread them over one month for example. Trying to do too much all in one go may put you off for life and that is the last thing I want you to do if you are gang to take control of your endometriosis!

CONSCIOUS EATING

*   **Shop online** This is great if you are strapped for time and can make it a lot easier to have the cupboards stocked with the foods you need to make the right choices.
*   **Delivery boxes** Think about signing up for a delivery box scheme near you. They deliver fresh and seasonal fruits and vegetables with recipe ideas on how to cook them as well as providing meat and other local and organic produce.
*   **Find your local good food 'dealer'** Find a source for local and organic vegetables and meat, either delivered to your door or at a convenient shop. You can always freeze stuff in advance. In the Useful Contacts section is a list of genuine organic box schemes (page 162).
*   **Discover your local health food store** Find a good health store near you where you can stock up on snacks such as nuts and seeds or healthy alternatives to junk-loaded snack food.
*   **Get machinery** Consider getting a blender and a bread machine. A blender will make cooking meals such as soups or smoothies so easy and practical. A very worthwhile investment. A bread machine will not only give you a great sense of satisfaction (or is that just me?) but it also allows you to make gluten-free loaves (if you need to avoid gluten) as much as you like without it costing a fortune. Ours is constantly on the go! We also have a juicer attachment that fits onto our food processor, which is a lot cheaper than buying a separate piece of equipment.
*   **Invest in a water filter** We have a water filter in our home that is plugged into the water system. It is expensive in the first instance but really does pay for itself and over a couple of years would be cheaper and more effective than using the jug-style filters. Our filter is from a company whose systems, put simply, take the nasties out and keep the goodies in. Other filters can take the nasties and the good minerals out too. See Useful Contacts, page 164, for more information.
*   **Get a steamer** Use this to cook all your vegetables rather than boiling them. This

way they retain their nutrient value more effectively. If you do not have a steamer you can make one by putting your colander over the top of an open saucepan, with a little boiling water in the bottom, and placing the lid over the top. As some of the goodness will have gone into the cooking water, you can use this for making soups.

- **Eat every three hours and don't skip meals** Going for long periods of time without food threatens your blood sugar balance and over time your hormone equilibrium. It also misses opportunities to feed your body's nutrients.
- **Pile on the fats** Eat plenty of foods rich in essential fats such as fresh salmon, mackerel, fresh tuna, nuts and seeds.
- **Cook with wonderful spices** Turmeric, ginger, rosemary, cumin, fennel and parsley have been shown to have benefits such as reducing inflammation and supporting digestion as well as making the food taste delicious.
- **Ease the stimulants** Cut down/out caffeine to twice per day, tops, if you can.
- **Get 'whole-y'** Chose wholegrain products rather than 'white' products.
- **Watch gluten** It is wise to ease up on gluten foods regardless of whether or not you have an intolerance or allergy. Our western diets do tend to include a lot of it and over time it can damage the gut wall and therefore general well-being.
- **Eat variety and in season** Make your plate colourful. When it comes to fruit and vegetables, the body was created to work in synergy with the natural habitat. Eating seasonally will provide the right nutrients, in the right order and at the right time.
- **H_2O** Aim for at least 1.5 litres of water per day but avoid drinking too much with meals as it can weaken digestion.
- **Keep lean protein in each meal** Include lean protein in each meal to enhance your energy levels and supports repair and manufacture of hormones. Combine with wholegrains.
- **Ditch the sugar** Substitute with organic dried fruit, and local or Manuka honey where you cannot do without a pinch of sweetness.
- **Get fruity (and veggie!)** Include a minimum of five *portions* each of fruit and vegetables every day and keep them varied. A great way to do this is by juicing or making compotes or curries.

* **Balance your hormones with plants** Pile on the pulses, tofu and green leafy vegetables to boost your intake of naturally occurring compounds that balance your oestrogen levels.

CONSCIOUS LIVING

* **Find ways to chill out** Look at ways to calm down your life where necessary. Do you need to go out more than twice a week? Do you have to work until 7.30pm every day? Is having a relaxing bath as beneficial for you as pounding a treadmill to release stress? Look at your priorities and work your life around them as much as you can.
* **Check your cooking utensils** Cooking apparatus made with aluminium can be associated with digestive system complaints ranging from mouth ulcers to piles. Non-stick Teflon coatings may also lead to gut trouble when they start to peel off.
* **Nutritional consultation?** If you think you have an intolerance or allergy book an appointment with a nutritional therapist who will help you to find the offending culprit.
* **Get moving** Find a way to exercise regularly in a way that is nourishing for your mind and body and that you will feel able to stick to in the long term.
* **Body brush** This is especially important for the Kickstart Cleanse (page 112) but is a great habit to get into once or twice a week to stimulate the circulation of nutrients and encourage the removal of toxins from the lymph system.
* **The 80/20 rule** Often we develop beliefs about 'good' or 'bad' foods. Some foods are 'good for us' even if we don't enjoy them. Other foods are 'bad for us' and we eat them guiltily or avoid them resentfully. If you have this attitude it is all too easy to feel you have failed by having one 'bad' day. Instead think of them as 'nourishing' or 'less nourishing' and whichever choice you make remember that it is *a choice* and accept the food with pleasure. Eat with the knowledge that by doing the things that nourish 80 per cent of the time, the rest of the time takes care of itself. This is the 80/20 rule. In this way we will get the most out of all foods.
* **Relaxation** The Chinese believe that it is better not to mix food and work. Our digestion works best when we are focused on our enjoyment of the meal, not distracted or troubled by other influences. So it is better to make mealtime a

relaxed occasion when we are not trying to read, watch television or work. So take the time to stop at lunch and at supper and enjoy the eating process.

- **Lose the tension around food** It is helpful to take a little time to relax our posture too, perhaps take a few quiet breaths before eating. Crossing our legs, sitting twisted or hunched will compress our digestive organs and hinder the passage of food through our body.
- **Shop 'loose'** Where you can, avoid packaging and if you cannot avoid doing so, take it off before you store your food.
- **Chew well** There is a saying: 'The stomach has no teeth'. Well-chewed food lessens the work our digestive organs have to do and increases the efficient extraction of nutrients. Chewing also warms chilled food.
- **Stop eating just before you are full** In a culture of plenty this can sometimes be difficult. If we overeat at any one meal, we create stagnation, a temporary queue of food waiting to be processed. As a result we feel tired while our energy is occupied digesting the excess food.
- **Think clean, think green** Choose household and personal health products free from toxic chemicals. Think, would you give them to or put them on a child?

CONSCIOUS EATING OUT AND ABOUT

- **Indian** Avoid creamy Korma dishes and stuffed naan breads, choosing instead chicken, fish or vegetarian dishes roasted in the tandoor, or *saag* (spinach) dishes.
- **Italian** Tuck into the minestrone soup, mixed salad, the *fagioli e tuna* (bean and pasta) or fish options. If you cannot resist a slice of the good old pizza, how about having a slice from someone else's plate – your table of course – to go with your salad.
- **Thai or Chinese** Tuck into *miang yuan* (soft spring rolls with prawn and fresh mint) to start or any of the grilled prawn dishes. Choose steamed rice or plain noodles rather than the special fried rice or Singapore noodle varieties. Choose prawn or chicken stir-fries rather than sweet and sour pork or Peking duck.
- **Local pub** Look for fish, lamb or chicken dishes on the menu – grilled or slow-

roasted rather than fried. Ask for a baked potato perhaps. Snack on olives and nuts (but not roasted nuts or peanuts).

- **Lunchtime sandwich bar** Go for vegetable-based soups, salads or jacket potatoes filled with tuna or hummus.

SHOPPING LIST FOR YOUR STORECUPBOARD

- Gluten-free pasta such as rice, corn or quinoa pasta
- Cold-pressed, extra virgin olive oil
- Rapeseed oil to cook with or 'Good Oil' (an oil from pure hempseed and rich in omega 3, 6 and 9)
- Gluten-free bread
- Rice cakes or gluten-free crackers
- Dried organic fruit (unnecessary preservatives are used in the non-organic form)
- Nut butters (try brands available from health food stores as they will contain little or no sugar)
- Wholegrain rice or wild basmati rice
- Seeds – such as sunflower or pumpkin
- Nuts – such brazil nuts, almonds and walnuts
- Organic unsalted butter
- Herbal teas – camomile, peppermint, fennel are all great for the digestive system
- Rooibos, a tea packed with antioxidants for healing and a great substitute for caffeinated black tea. Green tea is great to 'wean' yourself off coffee or tea if you have decided to give this up
- Pulses – chickpeas, lentils and cannellini beans are good for making sandwich or baked potato fillers or dips
- Spices and herbs – turmeric, ginger, rosemary, cumin, fennel and parsley
- Tamari – wheat-free soya sauce
- Gluten-free porridge
- Gluten-free muesli
- Quinoa

In the Useful Contacts section I have listed some companies that can fulfil your needs for all of the above.

FINAL WORD

It takes time to build up and care for good health – just as it does with any loving relationship. In order to do this we need the right building materials; we will not thrive and heal without a balanced and nutritious diet. With every health-conscious breath that you take, every meal you eat, every drink you swallow, you are literally building yourself back to the state of well-being you so deserve. This gives your body the equilibrium it needs to find the hormonal balance that has been disrupted by endometriosis, thereby helping to relieve symptoms such as pain and fatigue.

PART 3

THE KICKSTART

TAKE CONTROL – THE KICKSTART CLEANSE 6

I hope that the previous chapters have highlighted the fact that what you do and do not put into your body plays a fundamental role in achieving total wellness, and more importantly in achieving equilibrium for your hormones.

In the following we will explore the absolute need for a fully functioning detoxification system in order to strengthen your ability to heal and help relieve the symptoms of endometriosis. In my view any approach to endometriosis that does not cleanse and nurture this vital system is like building a house on sinking sand; it simply will not last. We first need to cleanse the body of all the factors that may slow down its ability to heal and repair and indeed may be exacerbating the condition and symptoms. Then we need to nurture it with the tools it needs to maintain a strong immune system, healthy hormone production and fully functioning detoxification system.

A cleansing diet is a good thing for many of us. The term 'detox' however has been mightily overused and can include anything from a few days on fruit to a month of fasting under medical supervision. It is the latter that deserves the term detox and it is imperative that anyone considering a proper 'detox' does so only once a comprehensive consultation has taken place with a qualified nutritionist and possibly undertakes the detox medical supervision. In the cases of advanced endometriosis a full detox programme can make the symptoms much worse if not correctly supervised or handled. A regular gentle cleanse is both preferable and essential.

A considerable number of the health plans you see in magazines and 'detox in 24 hours' books just don't give your body the time it needs for the good work to get started properly. They are not specifically designed to promote hormonal equilibrium. Through years of experience, research and passion, professionally and personally, I have tailored the following Kickstart Cleanse to give you the essential foundation stone on which to rebuild your health in a way that is practical and lasting. Let it encourage you to rest, listen to your body's own healing capacity and adopt nurturing habits that cherish hormonal well-being. The Nurture Diet in Part 2 will give you the tools and inspiration to develop the roots of hormonal equilibrium that have developed during this Kickstart Cleanse. Both stages will set up a way of remaining truly healthy, that you can control.

The benefits do not just stop at managing your experience of endometriosis. Following the recommendations in this chapter can greatly improve your immune defences, balance mood, and promote clear skin, healthy hair and nails, as well as digestive health.

WHY IT IS CRUCIAL TO LOVE YOUR LIVER

Your liver filters *everything* that travels through your bloodstream. This includes toxins from your food, skincare products, the air you breathe and anti-nutrient chemicals such as caffeine or alcohol. It also regulates the immune system by destroying old red and white cells, and allergic compounds and bacteria that may have escaped into the blood. But perhaps the most significant major function of the liver for women with endometriosis is the removal of used hormones from the blood. It does this by filtering the blood, breaking down the used hormones, packaging them up and sending them to the gut ready for excretion.

When your liver is firing on all cylinders it is central to your hormonal health, but most people subject it to unacceptable levels of toxins. This is not good news for women with endometriosis. If the liver is overworked by other functions such as high environmental toxin intake or a diet low in nutrients, it can fail to remove all components of oestrogen from the bloodstream when it should. Instead components of this hormone remain free to roam around the body once again, disrupting hormonal equilibrium and feeding endometrial patches.

Often we will not notice this process happening straight away and a healthy external appearance can hide a toxic burden for a long time. Symptoms of toxic overload include hormonal disruption and progression of hormonal disease, fatigue, poor skin or hormonal fluctuations that bring about increased cramps or premenstrual syndrome – you become, like so many, the walking or vertical 'unwell'. Plenty of us have just learnt to 'accept' it.

In this age of chemically polluted air, water, food and nutrient-poor diets, the liver becomes sluggish and has to work much harder, putting it in even greater need of nutritional support. Consciously or unconsciously we are putting a chemical load into our body every day; it is a symptom of the modern world. Sometimes the toxins are generated as a result of products that benefit us – fumes in the air from cars, buses or aeroplanes, or washing detergents or pesticides on tropical fruit that allow them to ripen at just the right time on the supermarket shelf. It is how we protect our body from the negative return of these lifestyle choices that is critically important for health.

The liver is a wonderfully intelligent organ and can regenerate given the right tools to cleanse and heal but it also needs to work in synergy with its fellow detoxification organs, the kidneys, skin, gut and lymphatic system. The liver requires these organs to be strong enough to handle the 'toxic' packages it sends to them for elimination. So supporting all of these organs as well as supplying a vast amount of nutrients and the chance to rest is the crux of the Kickstart Cleanse. It is a total body approach and the benefits will be comprehensive.

The kidneys and bladder work in unison with the liver. Your kidneys ensure you have the right amount of key minerals like potassium running through the system and remove those you don't want like salts, nitrogen and other chemicals. This filtered matter is then passed on to the bladder which then packages a nice stream of urine to excrete these rejects. During the Kickstart Cleanse you may find that your wee is a little smelly and this is likely to be the reason.

If the liver is overloaded by all it has to process, the kidneys are required to complete the job on its behalf. This is tricky as the kidneys are not strictly built to deal with this work. So the liver delegates a chunk of toxins over to the kidneys who then sub-delegate it to the bladder and consequently you are left with a build-up of toxic waste in your urinary tract. This becomes a breeding ground for yeast infections and other bacteria and regular urinary tract infections can occur.

THE KICKSTART CLEANSE

The primary purpose of the Kickstart Cleanse is to bring hormonal equilibrium back and pave the way for natural changes to occur. It is a fabulously effective approach to achieving lasting vitality and helping to alleviate the symptoms of any hormone-related conditions, especially endometriosis. It has been tried, tested, honed and tweaked to perfection. The recommended diet has been enriched with selected foods to reduce oestrogen dominance and support the natural cleansing process. Days 1–2 are the preparation period to lure your body gently into the cleanse. Days 3–4 focus on the nutrient power of fruit and vegetables to kickstart the liver's cleansing process. The fibre and nutrient content of these wonderful foods will also provide vital antioxidant nutrients to heal damage and fibre to cleanse the gut. Days 5–6 bring in hormone-promoting grains to stimulate bowel function and remove toxic products. Days 7–14 continue to arm your liver with the nutrients for regeneration and the gut with fibre-rich food. The eating plan also adds essential protein for repairing damage to cells and building hormones.

Throughout the diet it is crucial to keep hydrated at all times. This will clear the toxins from your system at a greater rate and ease the physical side effects. Remember to drink before you feel thirsty. If you are thirsty it means the body is already dehydrated. Aim for 1.5–2 litres of pure water, around six glasses a day. If you are buying water, opt for glass bottles rather than plastic ones. I also highly recommend the Kickstart Cleanse drink every morning about half an hour before your breakfast. This is a mug of warm water to which you have added a capful of apple cider vinegar and a spoonful of good quality honey (Manuka or local honey). This stimulates the gut and wakens the liver.

NB: Please do not do this cleanse if you are pregnant or trying to become pregnant as the foetus and placenta are highly sensitive to absorbing toxins within the system. If you are trying to become pregnant consider holding fire for a month whilst doing the cleanse and picking up where you left off afterwards. As the cleanse can optimise the function of the hormonal and reproductive system, fertility may be considerably boosted. Please also contact your medical supervisor if you are on medication.

The Kickstart Cleanse takes the principles of the Nurture Diet outlined in Chapter 3 and builds on them to encourage the cleansing process. Here they are summarised in bullet form to save you having to flick back a chapter if you have forgotten.

* Reduce stress
* Get some sleep
* Reduce your non-food toxic load
* Cut out alcohol
* Stub out the fags
* Reduce your saturated fat intake
* Eat variety
* Cut out sugar
* Read the label and go local and/or organic
* Drink plenty of pure water
* Experiment with a cleansing juice every day
* Start each morning with a mug of warm water, apple cider vinegar and Manuka or local honey
* Dry brush your skin in the morning (a must) and evening (if you remember); see page 120
* Gentle exercise after day 5

Days 1–2 Prepare your body by removing caffeine, alcohol, gluten and sugar from your diet. Drink mineral water, lightly steeped green tea or herbal teas. Eat large salads (warm salads of root vegetables, stir-fries or soups in the winter or colder weather) with beans, tofu, lentils or poached, grilled skinless chicken, turkey or fish. Fresh bean sprouts are intensely nourishing; grow your own or hunt them down in a health food store or forward-thinking supermarket. Add to salads or lightly stir-fried vegetable dishes, along with mixed seeds such as sunflower or pumpkin. Make wonderful dressings with cold-pressed olive oil, rapeseed oil, walnut oil, flaxseed or hemp oil. Drink plenty of water during the day, avoiding big slurps at mealtimes. The purpose of these two days is to prepare you and your body so that the changes are not too much of a shock to the system, easing you in gently.

Days 3–4 The Kickstart Cleanse steps up a notch now. This begins with a 48-hour period of just vegetables and fruit – juiced, stewed, baked, raw, dried or blended – however you prefer them but *not fried*. During the winter or colder weather eat as much of them warm as possible. One word of warning is that dried fruit contains concentrated levels of fructose and will make you very windy if you eat too much. It is about balance and the greater the range, the better for you. Fruit is easily digested and provides a wonderful amount of antioxidants that are needed to repair damage and for healing. Fruit also provides a wonderful source of fibre that feeds the good bacteria in the gut. Drink as much warm water with the juice of half a lemon as you can throughout the day. This is fabulous at balancing the pH of the body as well as encouraging the breakdown of toxic accumulation.

In these first few days you may feel a little tired and irritable (more than usual that is!), and develop a few spots, headaches or listlessness – not dissimilar to the feeling of a hangover. You may feel as though you are about to get your period with some mild cramping or even blood spotting. This is part of the liver's work on stabilising hormonal equilibrium as well as clearing excess inflammatory chemicals. For this reason it would be wise to schedule the start of the cleanse over a weekend so you can allow the process to happen a little more conveniently. Make sure you get plenty of pure water, herbal teas, fresh air, light and gentle amounts of exercise such as walking, yoga or similar. This is an energy-taxing time on the liver and needs to be respected as such, so go easy; no hardcore parties or very strenuous exercise. Some people find they get a little tearful or are quicker to anger – many natural health experts believe this is because the liver holds the emotion of anger. For those who are conditioned to repress anger, clearing the liver's garbage can also clear out stored emotions.

During this stage it is very, very easy to feel like giving up. Believe me I know it first-hand. I simply cannot emphasise the rewards you will reap for persevering. By taking this small period of time out of your life to empower your own self-healing you will feel a phenomenal difference, mentally, physically and emotionally.

If you think that candida is a problem for you then substitute the fruit for vegetables applying the same principles, so that you are eating just rice and veg from days 3–4. My strong belief that has been proven time and again in my clinic is that candida is a symptom not a disease and by cleansing the system you are in fact tackling the root cause of candida. Many who think they have candida can actually tolerate stewed fruits, so this is certainly worth a try.

Days 5–14 Now add in gluten-free wholegrain products from day 5 and lean proteins from day 7. Wholegrains that are gluten-free are quinoa and wholegrain rice (includes rice cake crackers). Lean proteins include veal, poultry and fish. For lunch and supper eat fresh salads and steamed, juiced, lightly stir-fried or slow-roasted vegetables. Use warm foods in the colder weather or if it is a damp day. Spice up the flavours with ginger, cardamom, cumin, fennel seed, turmeric, rosemary, chillies or garlic. Not only do these give extra flavour but they have wonderful health benefits too, including a proven ability to reduce inflammation and encourage digestion. During a cleanse I tend to crave these rich spices. Drink as much warm water with the juice of half a lemon as you can throughout the day.

You may begin to feel less 'toxic' at this stage and your energy should be improving. By day 10 you will be fully in the swing of the new regime and feeling the benefits. This is a fabulous way to continue your diet and is the very basis of the Stage 2 Nurture Diet. It redresses any excess acidity in the body caused by a sluggish detoxification system. As excess acidity leads to inflammation, the knock-on effect of reduction is obvious.

I really do encourage you to continue the 5–14 day plan for another 10–14 days if it is practical to do so. I find that after 10 days you have begun to feel great, but after 20–28 days you feel magical!

CLEANSE YOUR LIFESTYLE

Supplying nutritious food is not enough; you must also eliminate waste by reducing the amount of toxins you take in and by supporting the avenues by which they can leave. A lot of the body's waste products leave via the breath and skin. Therefore exercise, deep breathing and drinking plenty of water help cleanse the body and will support the effectiveness of the Kickstart Cleanse. This cleansing period is the golden opportunity to break less healthy habits and replace them with health promoting ones that you can continue for the long term.

- **Go organic** Removing as many chemicals and pesticides as you can from your diet is essential. Choosing organic fruits, vegetables and meat is vital. Organic produce contains more of the most valuable nutrients needed for hormonal balance such as minerals and essential fats.[1] Fruit, vegetables and meat are the priority if your budget is restricted. This is because the use of hormone-threatening pesticides is abundant in non-organic fruit and vegetables. If you cannot manage to eat all organic fruit then fruits with a 'peel' such as oranges or lemons can take a backseat. For vegetables, don't peel them if they are organic, they can just be scrubbed; the majority of the nutrients live immediately under the skin. As grains are very small they are able to absorb a lot of the chemicals thrown on them, so choosing organic forms can also make a vast difference. Animals reared non-organically can be fed a cocktail of antibiotics and hormones as well as food that has been sprayed with pesticides. As we know, the effect of xeno-oestrogens magnify and so by the time they reach us our consumption will be large. As you know from reading other sections of the book, adding this extra burden of synthetic oestrogens will contribute to the oestrogen dominance that already exists in women with endometriosis and potentially exacerbate the condition.
- **Drink pure water** This is covered in more detail in previous chapters but 'pure' properly filtered water makes a significant improvement to your toxic load. If you do not have a water filter system buy glass-bottled mineral water.
- **Cleanse skin-deep** As you will have already read, the skin is a major elimination organ for toxins. Part of encouraging it to do its job so well is being mindful about what we put on it. Use organic natural products that avoid the use of parabens and other xeno-oestrogens. For more detail on these see Keeping Clean and Green on page 174.
- **Exercise** Exercise is fantastic at getting the lymphatic system working, supplying nutrient-rich blood to the right organs. It also encourages the elimination of toxins through the skin by sweating. But during a cleanse energy needs to be preserved for healing, so go gently. It is a cliché but really do listen to your

body. If you are feeling tired, achy or in need of an early night don't pound the pavement in your trainers. Light exercise such as walking, yoga, Pilates, swimming or gentle jogging is better in the first few days.

- **Dry skin brush** Do this each morning or use an exfoliating mitt before you shower to get the circulation going. Skin brushing is a really effective way of shifting the lymphatic fluid and the toxins contained within it, and can be an effective technique in combating cellulite and promoting the cleanse. Ideally, brush dry skin for about 5 minutes once or twice a day. Brush quite vigorously but not enough to hurt, paying particular attention to the back of the legs and arms. Always brush in the direction of the heart to encourage the correct blood flow. This means you will be brushing upwards until the breast area and downwards or across for the upper torso.

- **Get steamy** If you have access to a hammam, sauna or steam room then use this, once or twice during the Kickstart Cleanse. This will encourage the elimination process. Make sure you are fully hydrated before and afterwards.

- **Take a long bath** Have a bath in Epsom salts. Epsom salts balance the pH level of the body. As you will see in the Nurture section of the programme, keeping a balanced pH level is crucial in reducing the inflamed areas in endometriosis.

- **Massage yourself** After your bath or shower massage in your body oil, especially around the chest and upper legs. As with dry skin brushing this will encourage the vital flow of lymph and support toxin removal.

- **Colonic irrigation** Colonic irrigation is complementary to any cleansing regime as it encourages the elimination of toxins that accumulate in the bowel. Colonic irrigation (also known as colonic hydrotherapy) is a treatment using water to stimulate and cleanse the bowel, aiding the evacuation of waste, and therefore toxic material that may have gathered in the bowel. If you decide to use this method I would advise booking an appointment for days 4–5 of the Kickstart Cleanse.

- **Chew each mouthful** Food serves not only as nourishment but also as a source of pleasure and stimulation. Take time over your meal and don't wash it down with drink. Saliva produced when you chew your food starts optimum digestion. It has the important job of breaking down the lumps of food and mixing it with enzymes in preparation for the stomach to do its job. If the food reaches the stomach without being broken down or chewed properly the stomach has to do double the work, which slows it down and makes it function less effectively. This then has a similar result in the intestines where all the vital nutrient absorption happens. If this part of the digestive process is compromised, so too is your nutrient supply. Your body's ability to produce the correct enzymes to break down food are particularly sensitive to stress so it is really important to relax before and after a meal.

◆ **Take a breath** This may sound trite but the importance of breathing properly and taking time to relax is vital in achieving maximum health. Breathing deeply, using the lower parts of the lungs (rather than the upper part, which the majority of people do), enables oxygen to circulate to the tissues, enriching them with nutrients and taking away waste. Deep breathing also stimulates the lymphatic system and induces a state of relaxation. Meditation, yoga, t'ai chi and qi gong all work on the breath, helping you to de-stress and taking the strain off the adrenal and pituitary glands that regulate hormonal balance. Often these glands are overworked in sufferers of endometriosis.

◆ **Get enough shut-eye** The body's most strenuous activity is ridding itself of undesirable substances. Each day a full 80 per cent of our energy is used on regenerating new cells for optimum detoxification. So this will be a taxing time for your system and you are likely to feel more tired as it gets to work. It is really important to respect your need for this. For the first few mornings you may wake up feeling you need to go back to sleep for another day and perhaps, where practical, this is what you should do. However, in the latter half of the cleanse you may feel like leaping out of bed with boundless energy.

◆ **Healthy cooking tips** Add herbs (rosemary, dill and chives), spices (cinnamon, turmeric, cardamom, fennel seed and cumin), lemon or garlic to add flavour to your food. The initial 'preparatory' days 1–2 are the best time to start bulk cooking stews, tagines, curries, soups and stewed fruit to keep in the freezer or fridge. This makes it that much easier to make the right choices when you arrive home hungry after work. There are now quite a few mail order companies that can deliver food to your door, whether at work or home, if you really don't have time to cook. A tiered steamer and a juicer are must-haves for any health conscious household and these are certainly worth investing in for the

Kickstart Cleanse and beyond. You can buy a juicer applicator to add on to a food processor if you have one of those already. Juicing and steaming retain significantly higher amounts of the nutrients found in fruit and vegetables, unlike boiling where the nutrients are leached out into the water. If you have to boil vegetables, the water can be used as a base for soups or stews. As nutrients are naturally degraded by heat, steam the veg or fruit for a couple of minutes until al dente, to preserve their nutrient provision. The slow cooking process used in stews and tagines is wonderful at preserving the nutrients in vegetables as they cook for longer but at a much lower heat. This process also gives a much tastier flavour without needing to use unnatural flavouring. Try to avoid fried or charcoal-grilled foods; although they give a lovely flavour they produce a high amount of compounds called free radicals that can damage cells and use up greater amounts of antioxidants. Try grilling or steam frying (by adding a small amount of water to a high heat).

If you are using non-organic fruit and veg, soak them in a bowl of water with a capful of organic cider vinegar to wash out the impurities or use a vegetable wash (a tasteless wash made from natural ingredients to remove farm chemicals, waxes, surface grimes or insects, available from most health food shops). If this isn't possible then peel the non-organic veg and fruit.

Think about getting rid of any cookware that is made of aluminium. As we discussed in the previous chapter, aluminium is a heavy metal, has serious health implications and is thought to contribute to the development of breast cancer. This has lead to it being classified as a metallo-estrogen, shown to mimic oestrogen in the body, thus activating oestrogen receptors. The same applies to aluminium foil. The best form of cookware is that made of cast iron, enamel, glass or stainless steel.

Avoid plastic wrapping (such as clingfilm) as much as possible. If you are buying foods from a supermarket take the fresh foods out of their plastic packaging as soon as you get home. Don't use clingfilm to wrap any fatty food such as cheese, and certainly don't heat anything in the plastic wrapping or containers as heat and fat within foods increases the amount of plasticisers or phthalates absorbed from the foodstuff's packaging. These synthetic chemicals are hard to remove from the body and can result in toxic build up, disrupting liver function and hormonal equilibrium.

FOODS TO EAT AND BUY WITH VIGOUR

The following foods are particularly brilliant at supporting the systems of elimination. Where possible choose in season.

KIDNEY	BLADDER	LIVER & GALLBLADDER	DIGESTIVE SYSTEM
Green peppers, Parsley, Watermelon, Endive, Dandelion, Grapefruit, Beetroot, Courgettes, Nettles, Cabbage, Lemon	Romaine lettuce, Onion, Mustard, Greens, Broccoli, Spinach, Blueberries, Parsley, Red Grapes, Lemon, Lettuce, Turnips, Oranges, Celery, Cabbage, Leeks, Dill, Lemon, Rhubarb	Apples, Carrots, Dandelion, Endive, Grapefruit, Lettuce, Parsley, Spinach, Tomatoes, Watercress, Chicory, Garlic, Onions, Rocket, Kale, Cabbage, Apricots, Radish, Strawberries, Sweet potatoes, Watercress, Asparagus, Brussels sprouts, Artichokes, Lemon, Turmeric, Eggs, Beetroot	Bok Choy, Beetroot, Onions, Apples, Garlic, Carrots, Dandelion, Endive, Grapefruit, Apricots, Artichokes, Brussel Sprouts, Fennel (and seeds), Celeriac, Dill, Mint, Tarragon, Turmeric, Pineapple, Papaya, Parsley, Ginger, Lemon, Rhubarb

Other foods to indulge in are:

- All fruit and vegetables not already listed
- Tamari (wheat-free soy sauce) – bit salty but great to add a little flavour
- Brown rice
- Corn
- Nuts
- Seeds

- Organic dried fruit (check sugar is not added)
- Seaweed (use with caution if on thyroid medication as iodine found in seaweed can interfere with these)
- Quinoa
- Marjoram
- Lean poultry
- Organic eggs
- Oily fish – mackerel, tuna, salmon and sardines from reliable sources
- White fish – halibut, pollack, dab and turbot

SUPPORTING THE KICKSTART CLEANSE WITH SUPPLEMENTS

It is especially important to support your detoxification system if you are doing a cleanse. Your body will be working hard to remove toxins from the body and in order to do this effectively it needs extra nutritional support. Without this the toxins that are being released in order to be removed can be reabsorbed into the bloodstream and cause damage.

In order to support any cleanse effectively you need a two-tiered approach. The first stage is to encourage the liver to clear the toxins and support the gut in eliminating them once it has done so. The second stage involves boosting the body with vital antioxidants to encourage healing of damaged cells and the production and regeneration of healthy cells and hormones.

I would encourage you to support this cleanse with a supplement regime formulated for cleansing. The following ingredients have been proven to support the cleansing and repair process particularly in hormonal conditions. Look for these ingredients in any products you choose. The supplement companies I recommend for these can be found in Further Help.

- **L-glutamine** An amino acid that is needed for the synthesis of rapidly dividing cells such as those lining the gut therefore aiding healing of the gut wall.
- **L-methionine** An amino acid responsible for protecting key liver compounds such as glutathione. Methionine is also responsible for 'de-activating' oestrogen

once it has been used for ovulation. Studies have shown methionine to improve liver function within six days.

- **N-acetyl cysteine** An amino acid needed for optimum liver clearing and reducing fatty build up in the liver that can cause it to become sluggish.
- **Dandelion root extract** Excellent at helping the liver to break down female hormones that have accumulated as a result of a sluggish liver. Don't confuse dandelion root with dandelion leaves that act on the kidneys.
- **Artichoke leaf extract** A herb to boost the regeneration of the liver cells. It also has a fabulous amount of protective compounds for defending the liver against damage.
- **Burdock root** Anti-inflammatory as well as a good blood cleanser. It also has an ability to protect the liver cells from damage associated with breaking down toxic matter in the bloodstream.
- **Milk thistle** (*Silybum marianum*) Contains a flavanoid called silymarin and is a truly excellent herb for generating new healthy liver cells to replace old ones. By effectively aiding the liver's capacity to break down excess amounts of oestrogen, it helps to balance the hormones.
- **Vitamin C** Enhances synthesis of glutathione as well as being a potent antioxidant, helping to repair damage caused by excess toxic load. Glutathione stores are used up when removing external toxins out of the system.
- **Alpha lipoic acid** A potent antioxidant that assists liver detoxification of pesticides and hormones.
- **Niacinamide (vitamin B3)** A member of the B vitamin family, this particular one is especially protective against damage to liver cells.
- **Bentonite clay** Acts as a sponge, binding to toxins, heavy metals and old hormones released into the gut allowing them to be flushed out of the system.
- **Apple pectin** A great source of fibre that, rather like bentonite clay, binds to toxins within the gut and removes them. It also helps to stabilise blood sugar levels.
- **Pyridoxine (Vitamin B6)** Essential for healthy liver function, proper digestion and absorption. B6 helps to de-activate oestrogen and render it harmless. Oestrogen does have a purpose and function within the body – we just don't want it in excess.
- **Beetroot** A rich source of fibre for gut cleansing as well as a rich source of iron.

- **Zinc** Essential for the immune system to work effectively and balance hormone production.
- **Chromium** To help stabilise blood sugar balance, generating the right amount of energy at the right time needed for damage repair.

FINAL WORD

By following the Kickstart Cleanse, you have taken the steps to teach, or re-teach, the body how to heal itself in a way that will set you up for a lifetime of health and vastly improve your experience of endometriosis.

I highly recommend undertaking the Kickstart Cleanse three times a year, September, February and May are my favourite times to do a cleanse. I choose end of January/beginning of February because I feel this is a gentler time of the year for the body. To do a cleanse at the beginning of January, straight after a time of festivities, can be quite harsh on your body after an indulgent period. I prefer to have a few weeks of rest and calm for the mind and the body so that the stage is set nicely for a gentle cleanse.

Our natural condition is to be healthy and therefore the ability to heal from disease is also natural. But in order for the body to heal itself, it needs a substantial amount of energy – otherwise we don't have the strength to stay healthy. Starting with a cleansed, restful system is the best starting ground for a healthy, healed body, giving your body the tools it will need to find hormonal equilibrium again and help to prevent the development and progression of endometriosis.

YOUR SAMPLE MENU AND RECIPES 7

Now you know what to eat and what not to eat on the Kickstart Cleanse but how do you go about it? Here are some ideas to help you plan the type of meals that will get you started with the dietary changes to help ease endometriosis.

SAMPLE MENU
Juices may make more than one glass so keep any excess in the fridge to drink throughout the day.

Each day on waking
Drink a mug of warm water to which you have added a capful of apple cider vinegar and a spoonful of Manuka honey. Wait 30 minutes, then have breakfast.

DAY 1
Breakfast
Mixed red berries (these can be frozen) such as blackberries, raspberries and blueberries whizzed or mixed with 3–4 tablespoons of live sheep's yogurt and a handful of mixed sesame, pumpkin and sunflower seeds. This combination is high in antioxidants, calcium and essential fatty acids.

Lunch
Steamed vegetables: sweet potatoes or squash, broccoli, cauliflower, carrots and green beans to make up 1–2 handfuls (depending on how hungry you are) of mixed veg served with brown rice. Make a sauce with fresh green herbs (mint, coriander and parsley) whizzed in a blender with two tablespoons of olive oil, the juice of half a lemon, a crushed garlic clove and a tablespoon of live yogurt. Add more olive oil if the dressing is too creamy. Sprinkle on some seeds.

Snack
Juice 1 celery, ½ cucumber, 1 apple, 1 pear and a 2cm peeled and chopped piece of ginger. This is fabulous for making the digestive environment more alkaline. To get the most health benefits out of it drink slowly, don't gulp.

Supper
Chicken breast with thyme and sage. Lightly sauté one chicken breast (weighing approx 250g and cut into small pieces) with one chopped spring onion for about 10 minutes until the chicken is lightly browned. Add 1 teaspoon each of chopped thyme, sage, lemon zest and coriander leaves. Serve with steamed carrots and green beans.

Juice of the day
Juice ½ papaya, a handful of red berries, ¼ cup of cranberries (½ teaspoon of cranberry powder if you can't get the fruit) and 2 apples. This juice is full of antioxidant power and a wonderful supporter of the liver and kidneys.

DAY 2
Breakfast
½ freshly grated apple and half a cup of chopped dried apricots with a teaspoon of ground cinnamon and 1 tablespoon of flaked or chopped almonds. Spoon over 3–4 tablespoons of live yogurt or porridge made with water or dairy-free milk such as soya or almond milk.

Lunch
'Sprouted seed' salad: Mix 2 handfuls of mixed sprouted seeds with some 2 tablespoons of stir-fried fermented tofu (if you like tofu!) or with the same amount of organic feta cheese and 1 tablespoon of chopped olives.

Supper
Grilled fish such as rainbow trout, Atlantic (organically farmed) salmon with 1 tablespoon of chopped mint, juice of half a lemon, chopped clove of garlic, 4 tablespoons of olive oil (mix all together in a bowl and serve on top of the fish). Serve with quinoa, courgettes and green beans.

Juice of the day
Juice 1 celery stalk, 2 apples and 1 carrot together. This is a great digestive tonic.

DAY 3
Breakfast
Mix together 4–5 de-stoned prunes, ½ banana and ½ pear with a tablespoon of mixed pumpkin seeds and walnuts. Add some live soya, goat's or sheep's yogurt to the mixture if desired.

Lunch
Baked sweet potato with hummus. Serve with a green salad, half a chopped avocado and 2 tablespoons of mixed sprouts dressed with garlic olive oil (infuse a peeled garlic clove in a small bottle of olive oil).

Supper
Warming Cauliflower Stew (see page 139).

Juice of the day
Juice 1 pear, ¼ grapefruit, 3cm peeled and chopped ginger and 1 teaspoon of Manuka honey. Water down with some apple juice (not from concentrate). This will help to boost blood circulation and encourage the delivery of nutrients around the body.

DAY 4
Breakfast
Smooth Berry Muesli (see page 135).

Lunch
Rocket, watercress and chicory salad sprinkled with mixed nuts and seeds (pine nuts, sesame seeds, walnuts) and an olive oil and lemon juice dressing.

Supper
Thai Vegetable Curry (see page 142) with steamed green beans and brown rice.

Juice of the day
Juice ½ pineapple, 2 tablespoons mixed blackberries, strawberries and blueberries, add water or yoghurt if too solid. This will help to improve circulation and reduce inflammation.

DAY 5
Breakfast
Chopped fruit such as ½ papaya, ½ mango, ½ passionfruit with a sprinkling of 1 teaspoon of ground cinnamon and 1–2 tablespoons of gluten-free muesli.

Lunch
Vegetable dip: carrot, celery, cucumber and chicory dipped in hummus (homemade or bought) with added cinnamon. Half an avocado with prawns and a drizzle of lemon juice.

Supper
Chicken fillets with a Cannellini Bean Purée (see page 142), steamed spinach and baked sweet potato.

Juice of the day
Juice ¼ beetroot, ½ lemon, 2 celery sticks, 2 carrots with a pinch of turmeric. This will help to boost the skin and cleanse the blood.

DAY 6
Breakfast
1 grilled beef tomato or 2 large grilled mushrooms on gluten-free bread with a little organic butter.

Lunch
Fresh, good quality vegetarian, salmon or tuna sushi of your choice with some edamame beans.

Supper

Polenta cooked according to the packet instructions with a garlic, tomato and basil sauce. Gently fry 1 chopped garlic clove and once this is golden add 200g chopped tomatoes, 1 tablespoon of balsamic vinegar and 1 tablespoon of chopped basil. Top with chopped organic feta or mozzarella.

Juice of the day

Juice 2 apples and ½ papaya with lemon zest from 1 lemon. To help the liver, kidney and provide antioxidants.

DAY 7

Breakfast

Chopped fruit of your choice, such as 1 apricot, 1 plum and ½ an apple served with 2 tablespoons of yoghurt or porridge.

Lunch

Mixed green leaves such as spinach, rocket and watercress served with 100g chopped goat's cheese and a tablespoon of chopped walnuts. Dress with olive oil and the juice of half a lemon.

Supper

Grilled Mackerel with Steamed Sweet Potato and Watercress (see page 140).

Juice of the day

Juice 100g tomatoes, 1 celery stick, ½ cabbage and 5cm peeled and chopped ginger. Add a dash of chilli powder and sip slowly. Detoxifies the liver, digestive tract and kidneys.

DAY 8
Breakfast
1 poached or scrambled egg on a slice of gluten-free bread.

Lunch
Celeriac Coleslaw with Prunes (see page 138).

Supper
Steamed Wild Trout with Puy Lentils and an Avocado Salad (see page 140).

Juice of the day
Beetroot Zinger (see pages 144–5).

DAY 9
Breakfast
Grilled Herb Tomatoes on Toast (see page 137).

Lunch
A Seasonal Vegetable and Fresh Herb Salad (see page 138).

Supper
Veal Meatballs with Grated Beetroot (see page 141).

Juice of the day
Apple Spice (see page 144).

DAY 10
Breakfast
Passionate Fruit Compote with fresh yogurt (see page 135).

Lunch
A Wholesome Salad with a Fresh Mint Dressing (see page 139).

Supper
Mixed herb omelette made using 1 tablespoon of basil and parsley, 1 cup of fresh spinach (half a cup of frozen spinach) and 1 chopped tomato. Served with steamed kale with a knob of butter and a squeeze of lemon.

Juice of the day
Carrot Zinger (see page 143).

RECIPES
I know that a change in cooking style can leave you stuck for ideas of what to cook, especially if you have not cooked with some of the recommended foods before. The following recipes have been designed by professional cook Louise Henkel to get you started. They are truly delicious and creative and can be used for both the Kickstart Cleanse and the Nurture Diet. Feel free to experiment with them, swap things if they don't appeal, add those that do from the 'Eat with Vigour' table (page 123) but keep the variety. The trick is be sure to plan ahead so that you are not tempted to grab something less healthy out of convenience. In general keep evening meals light and cooked to lighten the load on the digestive tract. All the following meals serve 1–2 people.

KICKSTART BREAKFAST IDEAS
Smooth Berry Muesli

100g mixed berries (e.g. raspberries, blackberries and redcurrants (can be frozen)

2 tablespoons sheep's yogurt
100g gluten-free muesli

Whizz the mixed berries and yogurt together in a food processor. Serve on a bowl of the muesli.

Winter Warmer with Porridge

1 apple, skin on, grated
thumb-size piece of ginger, grated
1 dessertspoon dried organic apricots, chopped

25g ground almonds
1 teaspoon cinnamon
80g gluten-free porridge oats cooked with 440ml of water

Serve the apple, ginger, apricots and ground almond with cinnamon sprinkled on porridge.

Passionate Fruit Compote

a handful of dried organic prunes, de-stoned
1 pear, chopped
1 banana, chopped

1 passionfruit, halved
a handful of pumpkin seeds
a handful of walnuts

Stew the prunes with pear in a saucepan over a low heat for about 10 minutes. Once cooked add the banana. Pour over the insides of the passionfruit and sprinkle with pumpkin seeds and walnuts.

Gooseberry and Almond Compote

100g gooseberries
1 tablespoon of honey

2 tablespoons ground almonds

Put the gooseberries into a saucepan with a tablespoon of water and the honey. Cook over a low heat, stirring occasionally, until the berries have become soft and stewed. Add more water as it cooks if necessary. Add the ground almonds, mix together and serve.

Cinnamon, Apple and Raisin Compote

30g raisins or sultanas
3 strips lemon zest
1 tablespoon of honey
1 small cinnamon stick, broken in half

150ml water
1 apple, sliced
juice of ½ lemon

Heat the raisins or sultanas, lemon zest, honey, cinnamon stick and water in a saucepan over a low heat until the mixture begins to blend together and become stewed. Meanwhile in a bowl mix the apple and lemon juice, and then add to the raisin mixture in the pan. Bring to the boil and simmer for about 5 minutes so that the apple is soft but still holds it shape. Take off the heat and leave to cool. I find the flavour of this compote develops if you cook it in advance and leave to cool in the fridge over night.

Serve all the above compotes warm or cold with a generous dollop of live organic yogurt (soya or goat's yogurt if avoiding cow's milk) or with gluten-free porridge. All can be made in advance in batches and frozen.

Grilled Herb Tomatoes on Toast

1–2 beef tomatoes

1 tablespoon white wine vinegar

2 tablespoons mixed herbs (such as
dried oregano, chives)

2 slices of gluten-free bread

butter

a handful of rocket leaves, chopped

Cut the tomato(es) in half. Grill cut-side down for 3–5 minutes (depending on the power of your grill). Turn so the cut-side is now facing up and add a drizzle of the vinegar and herbs and grill for the another 3–5 minutes. Lightly toast the bread, butter it, pop the tomatoes on top and sprinkle the rocket over the top.

LUNCH IDEAS (PORTABLE FOOD)

These are all quick, easy recipes that can be made in advance and will be popular with all of the family.

A Delicious Gluten-free Open Sandwich with Hummus

1 tablespoon organic or homemade
hummus per slice of bread

2–3 slices gluten-free bread per person

a handful of alfalfa seeds

Spread the hummus thickly on the bread and sprinkle with the alfalfa seeds. This is a simple, fast and delicious lunch that is very portable for work or eating on the go.

A Seasonal Vegetable and Fresh Herb Salad

150g asparagus
a handful of broad beans (if in season)
150g purple sprouting broccoli
50g garden peas, cooked
a handful of sprouted seeds

2 tablespoons mixed seasonal herbs
    such as mint, parsley, chives, basil
2–3 raspberries and blueberries
50ml extra virgin olive oil
juice of ½ lemon

Blanch or steam the asparagus, broad beans, purple sprouting broccoli and chill immediately. Add the cooked peas, sprouted seeds and herbs and mix well. Throw in the fruit just before eating to add some sweetness and colour – it will brighten up your day as you proudly unpack your delicious salad at work or simply on your own at home. Dress with extra virgin olive oil and lemon juice.

Celeriac Coleslaw with Prunes

1 small bulb celeriac, grated
1 apple, grated and tossed in approx
    1 tablespoon lemon juice
1 tablespoon mixed seeds such as
    pumpkin, poppy, sunflower

3 carrots (preferably organic), grated
2 tablespoons mixed herbs such as
    coriander, parsley and basil, chopped
    finely
a handful of dried prunes

For the dressing
2 tablespoons olive oil
1 teaspoon Dijon mustard

1 teaspoon sherry vinegar
juice of 1 orange

Mix together the dressing ingredients in a small bowl. Throw all the other ingredients into a bowl and then stir in the dressing. This can be kept in the fridge for up to three days. Eat on its own or with some steamed fish such as mackerel or sardines.

A Wholesome Salad with a Fresh Mint Dressing

25g mint

1 garlic clove, crushed

1 tablespoon olive oil

salt and freshly ground black pepper

100g red kidney beans, soaked overnight and cooked in plenty of boiling water

100g black-eyed beans, soaked and cooked

100g quinoa, simmered in 600ml water for 15 minutes

100g organic chickpeas, soaked and cooked

50g organic feta cheese, crumbled (optional)

If soaking and cooking your pulses is impractical for you, use organic tinned versions instead and rinse through.

Pulse together the mint, oil, garlic and seasoning in a food processor. You can also add a tablespoon of live yogurt if you wish. Mix together the cooked beans, quinoa and chickpeas in a serving bowl and stir in the mint dressing. Sprinkle the feta over the top.

Warming Cauliflower Stew

1 onion, finely chopped

1 leek, thinly sliced

1 celery stick, thinly sliced

½ small cauliflower, florets only

1 parsnip, peeled and finely diced

1 tablespoon fresh thyme, chopped

1 teaspoon fennel seeds

½ red chilli, finely chopped

600ml water

1 tablespoon honey

a pinch of white pepper

Maldon sea salt

Preheat oven to 180°C. Place the onion on a tray and bake in the oven for 30 minutes or until it starts to soften. Put all of the vegetables, including the baked onion, herbs and spices in a saucepan and cover with the water and honey. Bring to the boil and simmer for 15 minutes until tender. Season with pepper and salt. Either blend using an electric blender, adding some more water or fresh chicken stock and fresh thyme leaves, or enjoy the rustic nature of a hearty textured soup.

SUPPER IDEAS

Grilled Mackerel with Steamed Sweet Potato and Watercress

2 sweet potatoes, chopped
1 mackerel, filleted
Maldon sea salt and black pepper
150g fine green beans

50g watercress
1 handful skinned almonds
1 garlic clove, crushed
2 tablespoons Good Oil or other
    omega oil

Steam the sweet potatoes for 25–30 minutes. Meanwhile season the mackerel and grill skin-side up for approximately 3 minutes until cooked (the flesh should come away easily from the skin). Add the green beans to the steamer for the last 5 minutes, on top of the sweet potatoes. Remove the sweet potatoes from the steamer and crush/ mash with a fork. Chop the watercress, almonds and garlic and mix with the potatoes. Stir in the oil and season. Serve the mackerel on top of the mashed sweet potato with the fine green beans on the side and season with salt and pepper.

Steamed Wild Trout with Puy Lentils and an Avocado Salad

2 x 175g wild trout fillets
1 tablespoon fresh ginger, julienned
½ lime, sliced

1 red chilli, julienned
20g fresh coriander, chopped
100g ready-prepared Puy lentils

For the salad
1 avocado, cubed
1 cucumber, cubed

2 spring onions, chopped

For the dressing
15g dill, finely chopped
1 garlic clove, crushed
1 teaspoon water

1 tablespoon lime juice
1 teaspoon honey

Place the trout in a steamer with the ginger and lime and steam for approximately 8 minutes. Remove from the steamer and sprinkle the chilli and fresh coriander on top. Mix the ingredients for the dressing together in a small bowl. Add the salad ingredients and mix with the dressing. Serve the trout on top of the Puy lentils with the salad on the side.

Veal Meatballs with Grated Beetroot

For the meatballs

250g veal, minced

1 chilli, chopped

1 teaspoon ground cumin

1 egg, lightly beaten

2 tablespoons chopped parsley and
  coriander

1 beetroot, grated

1 garlic clove, crushed

1 teaspoon paprika

25g gluten-free breadcrumbs

salt and black pepper

For the sauce

200g small cherry tomatoes (whole)

1 red pepper (chop and remove seeds
  and stalk)

1 red onion, roughly chopped

a handful of basil, chopped

Preheat oven to 200°C. Roast the tomatoes, pepper and onion in the oven for 25 minutes. Leave to cool. Meanwhile, combine all of the meatball ingredients together in a mixing bowl using a fork and season with salt and pepper. Roll the mixture into golf-ball-sized meatballs and place them on a baking tray. Bake in the oven for 10 minutes. Remove the stalk from the pepper and pulse together with the tomatoes and onion in a food processor. Transfer to a saucepan over a low heat and then add the meatballs to the sauce and cook for 5 minutes on a low heat. Serve the chopped basil on top. Delicious served with brown rice and steamed cabbage.

Chicken Fillets with a Cannellini Bean Purée

2 chicken breast or thigh fillets,
    weighing about 250g
300ml fresh organic chicken stock
200g organic cannellini beans, soaked
    and cooked as per instructions

2 garlic cloves
juice of ½ a lemon
a handful of freshly chopped parsley

Poach the chicken fillets in the chicken stock for approximately 20 minutes (depending on their size). Pulse the cannellini beans, garlic and lemon juice together in a food processor and slowly add the chicken stock until you have the desired consistency – like a smooth hummus. Season and pour over the cooked chicken fillet and sprinkle with fresh parsley. Delicious served with sautéed leeks and roasted cherry tomatoes.

Thai Vegetable Curry

20g fresh ginger chopped
2 red chillies, chopped
2 sticks lemongrass, finely chopped
2 garlic cloves
1 teaspoon turmeric
2 shallots
1 dessertspoon rapeseed oil

250g diced root vegetables (a mixture
    of carrot, pumpkin, sweet potato)
1 x 400g can coconut milk
1 tablespoon Thai fish sauce
juice of 1 lime
2 teaspoons freshly chopped coriander

Sauté the ginger, chilli, lemongrass, garlic, turmeric and shallots in the oil. Add the vegetables and then slowly add the coconut milk and simmer for approximately 5 minutes. Season with Thai fish sauce, lime juice and coriander. Serve on brown rice.

KICKSTART CLEANSE JUICES

Juices are a great way to boost your nutrient and fluid intake. They also make great filling snacks during the day. They are easy for the body to assimilate quickly and efficiently, taking only 10–15 minutes to digest. Invest in a juicer or a versatile food processor, which allows you to experiment with different fruits and vegetables. It is best to combine vegetable juices. If the juice is too strong, dilute with a little mineral water. For a more filling juice you could add protein such as silken tofu, soya milk or yogurt – all organic where possible. Experiment and see which ones suit your taste.

All the following juice recipes make about 2 large glasses.

Carrot Zinger

The zing of the orange will boost energy and provide the antioxidant vitamin C. Carrots are excellent sources of minerals and encourage liver cleansing. Ginger will boost nutrient delivery in the blood. Sesame is rich in iron, which is crucial for energy. The combination will give your immune system a nutrient boost.

3 carrots, tops and bottoms removed
1 apple, cored and sliced
1 cm piece of fresh ginger (or more or less
   depending on how much of a kick you
   want to give it)

1 orange, peeled
1 teaspoon sesame seeds

Juice the carrots, apple, ginger and orange in a juicer. Stir in the sesame seeds and drink.

Apple Spice

Pectin, found in apples, is a great cleanser and remains in the juice after juicing. This also helps to balance blood sugar levels. Celery is also a potent cleanser and lemon helps to neutralise acidity.

3 apples, cored and quartered
3 sticks of celery

a squeeze of lemon juice

Juice the apples and celery, transfer to a blender, add the lemon juice and blend. Strain through a sieve. Serve warm or cold.

Avocado Ice

This is a drink rich in omega fats and vitamin E to help reduce inflammation. The lettuce and cucumber will encourage the elimination of toxins through the bladder and kidneys.

$\frac{1}{4}$ iceberg lettuce
1 lime
$\frac{1}{4}$ cucumber

$\frac{1}{2}$ avocado, peeled and stoned
1 teaspoon wasabi
3 ice cubes (optional)

Juice the lettuce with the lime and cucumber. Transfer to a blender and blend with the avocado, wasabi and ice cubes.

Beetroot Zinger

Beetroot is well known for its liver and blood cleansing properties. It contains a compound called salicylic acid (from which aspirin originates) that may help to combat the headaches that result from cleansing. It is also rich in iron, and the vitamin C in the orange encourages the absorption of this nutrient. Ginger is calming on the digestive tract and carrots contain the necessary antioxidants for repairing free radical damage associated with toxin overload.

2 beetroots, leaves left on
2 carrots, tops and bottoms removed

0.5cm piece of fresh ginger
1 orange, peeled

Juice all the ingredients in a juicer and stir to combine.

Clear Zing

The acid in the lime helps to ensure that the energy from the raspberry and orange juice is absorbed steadily, giving a gentle rise in blood sugar levels. The mint contains compounds that are great for relaxing the muscles of the digestive system and relieving symptoms of irritable bowel syndrome and trapped gas.

3 handfuls of raspberries
1 lime
2 oranges, peeled

6 mint leaves
3 ice cubes

Juice the raspberries, lime and oranges together. Chop the mint finely and combine. Pour over the ice cubes.

BASIC TIPS ON JUICES: Carrot will go with any fruit and apple will go with any vegetable. Drink juices within 30 minutes of making to get the optimum amount of nutrients and enzymes from the fruit or veg, or store in the fridge.

PART 4

WHOLE BODY
BENEFITS

HOW THIS APPROACH WILL NURTURE OTHER PARTS OF YOUR BODY

8

NURTURING YOUR FERTILITY

There is much fear around the subject of endometriosis and fertility, both among sufferers and health professionals. From years of feedback from women who have consulted professionals about their endometriosis, I have found too many have been left feeling disempowered and ultimately resigned to the idea that they will not be able to conceive naturally. I know this both as a practitioner and because I, too, have been on the receiving end of such news. However, I feel it is extremely important here to distinguish between infertility and sub-fertility. Infertility is a medical diagnosis given to couples who have tried to conceive naturally for some time, usually more than 12 months. Most will have tried natural lifestyle changes to enhance their fertility, undergone the relevant tests and have had no success as yet. They might have a very real physical obstacle such as a removed ovary or blocked fallopian tubes.

Sub-fertility, on the other hand means that a couple are on a back-foot in terms of fertility. They may not be in a state of optimum fertility but conception is potentially achievable through changes to diet and lifestyle and medical intervention such as surgical procedures to remove endometriosis for example.

Infertility is used too often as an umbrella term for any challenges to optimum fertility, often to the woman herself. This gives her the wrong impression about her ability to conceive and can set up a feeling of defeat and increased tension, which can contribute to blocking conception, creating a self-fulfilling prophecy.

SO DOES ENDOMETRIOSIS AFFECT YOUR FERTILITY?

The answer is yes and no. Some women will not be able to conceive naturally and statistics show that 30 per cent of these have endometriosis. However, endometriosis is a highly under-diagnosed condition and many women with the condition achieve healthy pregnancies without even knowing they have the endometriosis.

Fertility is a complex and multi-faceted process and is not guaranteed in any woman, but it can be made harder with endometriosis. Other factors involved include the quality of a man's sperm, age (of both partners), ovulation cycle, not to mention a relaxed state of mind, to name but a few. If you are experiencing problems conceiving it is these factors that need to be addressed as much as anything else, so please do not feel the onus is solely on you as the woman, or your endometriosis.

When you have decided you would like to become pregnant, you may start to notice every pregnant woman and baby as you walk down the street. It can become all-consuming. Every month that goes by can feel like you are one month further from being able to become pregnant. I cannot stress enough how far from the truth this is. The likelihood of becoming pregnant within the first month of intercourse without contraception is actually only 20 per cent, i.e., one couple in every five, for all couples. With every month that goes by where pregnancy may not have occurred, you could in fact be one month closer to when it does.

If adhesions of endometriosis are present in the fallopian tubes and/or ovaries this can prevent the transportation of the egg after ovulation. These adhesions stick the ovary or the fallopian tube to other tissue in the surrounding area. This can cause a 'kink' or even a blockage in the fallopian tube and make it hard for the egg to travel into the womb for implantation. Sometimes this is tested during surgery where dye is passed through the tube to see if it flows. Some women have their fallopian tubes 'flushed' and this has been shown to improve fertility.[1]

Having a laparoscopy to remove an adhesion can be a very successful way of rectifying the problem, and allowing 'free flow' again. Clinical evidence also shows that surgery to remove adhesions or endometrial patches achieves better results in improving the rate of pregnancy than any other conventional treatment.[2] If the adhesions are left and not supported with dietary management to control them, they may form chocolate cysts, which in turn can hinder effective ovulation.

Evidence suggests that medical hormonal treatment following laparoscopic surgery does not improve chances of pregnancy.[3] Research also shows the greatest chance of pregnancy is within 15 months of surgical treatment with laparoscopy.[4,5]

Pregnancy also needs a healthy supply of progesterone. Progesterone promotes the growth and protection of the fertilised egg (now an embryo). In other words it is needed to 'hold' a pregnancy. As women with endometriosis have a deficiency of progesterone because of the dominance in oestrogen this can also make the journey to pregnancy harder.

Women with endometriosis have weakened immune systems. This may cause a hostile environment for the survival and development of the embryo in early pregnancy.[6] We are sophisticated machines and, in terms of evolution, the fittest really do survive. We may be designed to conceive only when we are physically and mentally strong.

The thyroid gland and its hormonal products play a vital role in our overall well-being. The main hormone produced by the thyroid is thyroxine. Oestrogen is an antagonist to thyroxine; in other words it competes with thyroxine. Therefore a dominance in oestrogen easily results in poor thyroxine levels which can lead to thyroid conditions such as hypothyroidism (an underactive thyroid).

Another potential obstacle is that sex may be uncomfortable because of the inflammation and physical changes endometriosis can create internally which may, understandably, affect the frequency of intercourse. This should not be underestimated. It can be a contributory factor in lengthening the time it takes to become pregnant. If you find intercourse uncomfortable then other forms of intimacy that do not involve penetration can work just as well to unite you and your partner emotionally. But intercourse is needed to achieve pregnancy.

The nurturing way of life detailed in this book can contribute to your fertility greatly by avoiding environmental threats to hormone balance such as xeno-estrogens and promoting your reproductive functions with nutrient-dense foods. In essence the nature of the relationship between endometriosis and infertility remains unsolved. The balance of the evidence is that, apart from mechanical damage, endometriosis does not cause infertility.[7] Sub-fertility is a *symptom* of endometriosis. By adopting a nurturing way of living with supplements, reducing your toxin intake and eating to take control of your endometriosis you are also greatly improving your chances of fertility. By eating regular meals, avoiding saturated fat and sugars, boosting your intake of nutrient-dense foods, you can go a long way to managing inflammation, supporting hormonal equilibrium and strengthening the detoxification system. These are all factors that are integral for healthy fertility and can make a real difference whilst you are in the pre-conception stage. Your recommended supplements take this to another level still. Magnesium, vitamin B6 and vitamin E boost progesterone levels vital to protect the fertilised egg. Once you are pregnant I recommend you take a supplement programme specific to supporting the three trimesters of pregnancy.

If you have not become pregnant after 12 months of trying it would be a good idea to chat to your GP and perhaps undergo some preliminary tests to rule out anything preventing a pregnancy. If you feel you are finding it hard to wait that long, acupuncture or homeopathy can help you to mentally and emotionally relax.

PROTECT YOUR FUTURE HEALTH

As endometriosis is a condition fuelled by a dominance of oestrogen and a weakened immune system, it shares the physiological characteristics of female cancers.[8] Certain types of breast cancer and ovarian cancer appear to be triggered by high levels of oestrogen. So too does endometriosis. This is not to say that women with endometriosis go on to develop cancer but it seems that the lifestyle and genetic factors that are now known to influence the progression of endometriosis are those that also contribute to the development of breast and ovarian cancer.

More research is needed to look at the links between the development of the two diseases, cancer and endometriosis.[9] By improving health through a nourishing diet and lifestyle you can balance your hormonal system, strengthen your immune defences against damage and support the toxin elimination processes. By supporting the body in this way, you are doing much to counteract the risk.

Oestrogen is an umbrella term for three types of oestrogen in a woman's body. Two are likely to have the potential to cause cancer – oestradial and oestrone. The third – oestriol – is protective against cancer. Oestriol is the type of oestrogen formed in the liver from the oestradial and oestrone that is being cleared from the bloodstream. This is even more reason to support the health of your liver.

ENDOMETRIOSIS AND FIBROIDS

Fibroids are an overgrowth of the middle, muscular layer of the womb. They are oestrogen sensitive and can cause a great deal of swelling and pain. Some women with endometriosis develop fibroids and vice versa. This is probably to do with the dominance of oestrogen and the reduced ability of the body to control this. There is no link more significant than that. The nutrients and the dietary approach needed for managing fibroids are the same as those needed for endometriosis, so if you are experiencing both these conditions you will be hitting two birds with one stone.

FINAL WORD

No matter what we've been through or how bad we feel, we are always in a position to help ourselves reach wellness – to begin the healing process by taking responsibility for our lives and health. Making changes to your daily diet will give you the opportunity to take an active role in your experience of endometriosis. It will also means that you are taking significant steps to enhance your fertility, and future health, supporting your body's prevention of other related diseases such as fibroids and cancer. I hope that the information in this chapter, and those preceding it have provided you with the knowledge and encouragement to make this happen.

Taking stock of your lifestyle; looking at how you manage stress both internal and environmental, how much you exercise, looking after your emotional health and becoming aware of the ingredients in products you put on your body each day, means that you can play an active role in managing your endometriosis. The result being that you *take control of your endometriosis*, rather than it taking control of *you*.

PART 5

FURTHER HELP

APPENDIX 1: GLOSSARY

ablation A surgical procedure used to remove (ablate) endometrial tissue.

adhesions The medical term for patches of endometriosis. They can cause some of the organs to stick together and create a 'tugging' effect and subsequent pain.

anti-nutrients Food and products that use up more energy and nutrients from the body than they provide.

cervix The lower, narrow part of the womb (uterus) where it joins the top of the vagina.

cortisol A hormone produced by the adrenal gland when the body is under stress. Its primary functions are to increase blood sugar, suppress the immune system and aid in fat, protein and carbohydrate metabolism.

cul-de-sac The space behind the womb, also known as the pouch of Douglas.

diathermy Intense heat used in laparoscopy to remove or burn away patches of endometriosis.

dysbiosis A microbial imbalance on or within the body. This most prominently occurs in the digestive tract where good bacteria have lost the battle against bad bacteria.

dysmenorrhoea Pain during menstruation that interferes with daily activities.

dyspareunia Pain during sexual intercourse.

endometrial tissue Tissue from the womb (endometrium) that can appear elsewhere in the body (endometriosis), most commonly the lower part of the pelvis.

endometrioma Also known as 'chocolate cysts', they are larger lumps of endometriosis that grow inside the ovaries. They are filled with old blood hence their dark brown appearance.

endorphins Chemicals released by the brain that act as neurotransmitters and can relieve pain and produce a feeling of well-being.

enzyme A protein that increases a chemical reaction, for instance digestive enzymes are produced by the body to help break down food.

fallopian tubes The tubes in the female reproductive system that lead from the ovaries to the womb and allow the passage of eggs from the former to the latter.

gastrointestinal tract The stomach and intestine where the body's absorption of nutrients from food takes place.

gut motility (or gastric motility) The spontaneous movements of the stomach to aid digestion.

hysterectomy The surgical removal of the womb, which can sometimes include the removal of the ovaries and can be used as a treatment for endometriosis.

laparoscopy A medical investigative procedure that involves placing a laparoscope (an instrument through which structures within the abdomen and pelvis can be seen) through an incision in the navel to see if there are any abnormalities, such as endometriosis.

metaplasia A reversible change from a normal cell structure into an abnormal one, according to the cell's environment.

myalgic encephalitis (ME) Also known as chronic fatigue syndrome it is a condition that causes extreme tiredness.

oestrogen The female sex hormone secreted by the ovaries.

osteoporosis A disease occurring when the rate of bone renewal does not keep up with the rate of its breakdown, resulting in bones that are filled with tiny pores or holes.

ovaries Female reproductive organs that produce eggs for reproduction and the hormones oestrogen, testosterone and progesterone.

ovulation A process that occurs during the menstrual cycle where a mature egg is released from the ovary for possible fertilisation.

peritoneum A layer of cells, blood vessels and a lymphatic capillary network that covers the abdominal and pelvic walls and organs.

progesterone A hormone manufactured in the ovaries and adrenal glands that promotes the growth of the lining of the womb during the last half of the menstrual cycle. It enhances mood, helps protect against certain cancers and reduces (or stops) bone loss.

prostaglandins Hormone-like substances that participate in a wide-range of bodily functions such as the dilation and constriction of blood vessels, control of blood pressure and modulation of inflammation.

retrograde menstruation Also known as 'transplantation theory' this concept proposes that endometriosis is due to endometrial tissue abnormally flowing up the fallopian tubes in the blood and into the abdomen or bowel.

serotonin A chemical produced by the brain that functions as a neurotransmitter and is known for making you feel good.

stem cell One of the body's master cells with the ability to continuously divide and develop into more than 200 cell types.

testosterone A hormone produced by the ovaries and adrenal glands in women.

uteroscacral ligaments The ligaments connecting the sacrum and the cervix.

uterus Also known as the womb, this female reproductive organ is located between the cervix (opening into the vagina) and the fallopian tubes and is where the foetus develops during pregnancy.

xeno-oestrogens Synthetic industrial chemicals found in pesticides, fuels and drugs that cause hormonal activity similar to oestrogen and may alter the natural form of the hormone made by the body.

APPENDIX 2: USEFUL CONTACTS

SUPPLEMENT BRANDS

HenriettaNorton
www.henriettanorton.com
info@henriettanorton.com

BioKult
www.protexin.com
Email: info@protexin.com
Tel: 0800 328 5663

New Chapter
www.newchapter.com
Email: info@newchapter.com

Specialist Herbal Supplies
www.shs100.com
Email: moc.001shs@selas
Tel: 0845 053 5433

Natural Dispensary
www.naturaldispensary.co.uk
Tel: 01453 7577792

Nutri-centre
www.nutricentre.com
Tel: 0208 752 8450

Revital
www.revital.com
Email: enquire@revital.com
Tel: 0870 366 5729

HEALTH FOOD STORES

Wholefoods
www.wholefoodsmarket.com

Infinity Foods
www.infinityfoods.co.uk

Planet Organic
www.planetorganic.com

ONLINE ORGANIC DELIVERY

Riverford
www.riverford.co.uk

Find Local Produce
www.findlocalproduce.co.uk

Abel & Cole
www.abelandcole.co.uk

If you live outside a city check your area for local delivery schemes.

SUPPORT NETWORKS

Endometriosis UK
www.endometriosis-uk.org
Email: admin@endometriosis-uk.org
Tel: 0808 808 2227

The Endometriosis SHE Trust (UK)
www.shetrust.org
Email: shetrust@shetrust.org.uk
Tel: 08707 743665

Foresight preconceptual care
www.foresight-preconception.org.uk
Email: emailus@foresight-preconception.org.uk
Tel: 01243 868001

Infertility Network UK
www.infertilitynetworkuk.com
Tel: 0800 008 7464
Women's health
www.womens-health.co.uk
Women's Environmental Network
www.wen.org.uk
Email: info@wen.org.uk
Tel: 020 7481 9004
International Federation of Organic Agriculture Movements
www.ifoam.org
Tel: +49 (0)228 926 5010

HERBALISTS
National Institute of Medical Herbalists
www.nimh.org.uk
E-mail: info@nimh.org.uk
Tel: 01392 426022
Michael McIntyre
Midsummer Clinic
www.midsummerclinic.co.uk
01993 830 419

NUTRITIONAL THERAPISTS
Henrietta Norton Clinic
www.henriettanorton.com
Email: henrietta@henriettanorton.com
Clinics in London and Sussex

British Association of Nutritionists (BANT)
www.bant.org.uk
Email: theadministrator@bant.org.uk
Tel: 08706 061284

MEDITATION
British Meditation Society
http://www.britishmeditationsociety.org
Transcendental Meditation
http://www.tm.org/
London Shambhala Meditation Centre
http://www.shambhala.org.uk/

ACUPUNCTURE
The British Acupuncture Council
Tel: 0208 735 0400
Emma Cannon
A Healthy Conception
www.ahealthyconception.co.uk
Email: emma@emmacannon.co.uk
Yvonne Darnell
Unity Acupuncture Practice
www.unityfertility.co.uk
Email: info@unityfertility.co.uk
Tel: 01444 235400

ELECTROMAGNETIC STRESS ASSESSMENT
Roy Riggs
www.royriggs.co.uk
Email: roy.riggs@ntlworld.com
Tel: +44 01273 732523

YOGA
British Wheel of Yoga
www.bwy.org.uk
BWY Central Office
British Wheel of Yoga
25 Jermyn Street
Sleaford
Lincolnshire
NG34 7RU
Tel: 01529 306851
Biomedical Trust
31 Dagmar Road
London
N22 7RT
www.yogatherapy.org
Email: enquiries@yogatherapy.org

WATER FILTER COMPANIES
East Midlands Water
2 Cannock Street
Leicester
LE4 9HR
www.eastmidlandswater.com
Tel: 0116 276 3334
Freshly Squeezed Water
Freshly Squeezed Water Systems Ltd
PO Box 2208
Wolverhampton
WV3 8YD
Tel: 0844 873 3148

MEDICALLY SUPERVISED DETOX
The Breakspear Hospital
www.breakspearmedical.com
Email: info@breakspearmedical.com
Tel: 01442 261 333
The Mayr Clinic, Austria
www.viva-mayr.com
Quit Smoking
www.quit.org
Tel: 0800 00 22 00

SPECIALIST FOODS
Goodness Direct
www.goodnessdirect.co.uk
Tel: 0871 871 6611
Healthy, fresh, eco and organic foods
delivered to your door.
Sustainable Fish Guide
www.goodfishguide.co.uk
Raw Vibrant Health Living
www.rawhealth.uk.com
Organic raw ingredients that are mostly
soaked and sprouted for extra nutrients.
Lovely, health conscious snacks. Find
their stockists online.

GLUTEN- AND DAIRY-FREE
Amy's Kitchen
www.amyskitchen.co.uk
Provides great food for people that
need to use prepared foods. Home
cooked gluten-free, dairy-free food. All
ingredients are grown without the use of
organophosphate pesticides.

GLUTEN FREE
Kent & Fraser
www.kentandfraser.com
Tel: 0844 8404250
Sussex-based producers of delicious
gluten-free biscuits, savoury and sweet.
Sadly I had to research the entire range!
Amisa
www.amisa.co.uk
A range of delicious, extremely healthy
snacks, cereals and brands that are
gluten-free.
Hale & Hearty
www.halenhearty.co.uk
Tel: 020 7616 8427
The WAGfree Bakery
www.wagfreefood.com
Tel: 020 7274 6267
Leaveitout
www.leaveitout.co.uk
Food-allergy and gluten-free discounts
as well as specialist eating out guide.

BESPOKE CATERING FOR THOSE WITH PARTICULAR DIETARY REQUIREMENTS
Louise's Kitchen
www.lkitchen.co.uk
Email: louiseskitchen@fsmail.net
Cooking workshops for learning how to
embrace particular dietary needs.
In the Pink Cookery
www.inthepinkcookery.co.uk
Tel: 01225 743386

RAW MILK
Hook Dairy
www.hookandson.co.uk
Tel: 01323 449494
Plaw Hatch Farm
www.tablehurstandplawhatch.co.uk
Tel: 01342 810201

ORGANIC BODY CARE
Suti
www.suti.co.uk
Email: hello@suti.co.uk
Pia Skin Care LTD
www.paiskincare.com
Email: info@paiskincare.com
Tel: 0208 994 4656
Yes Baby Organic Lubricants
www.yesyesyes.org
Email: isis@yesyesyes.org
Tel: 0845 094 1141

Green People
www.greenpeople.co.uk
Email: organic@greenpeople.co.uk
Tel: 01403 740350

The Organic Pharmacy
www.theorganicpharmacy.com
Email: info@theorganicpharmacy.com
Tel: 0844 800 8399

PERSONAL HYGIENE PRODUCTS

Natracare
www.natracare.com

TOXIN-FREE HOUSEHOLD PRODUCTS

Earth Friendly
www.ecos.com
Email: contact@ecos.com

Ecover
www.ecover.com
Email: info@ecovercareline.co.uk
Tel: 08451 302230

Ecozone
www.ecozone.com
Email: eco.trade@ecozone.co.uk
Tel: 0845 230 4200

If you care
www.ifyoucare.com

Method
www.methodproducts.co.uk
Email: talkclean@methodproducts.co.uk
Tel: 0207 788 7904

OTHER

Plasma Surgical
For more information on Plasmajet surgery
www.plasmasurgical.com

FURTHER READING

HOLISTIC HEALTH

You Don't Have to Feel Unwell by Robin Bottomley (New Leaf, 1994)
Potatoes Not Prozac: How to Control Depression, Food Cravings and Weight Gain by Kathleen Desmaisons (Pocket Books, 2008)
The Self-Healing Human by Susanna Ehdin (Holistic Wellness Publication, 2003)
Fats that Heal, Fats that Kill by Udo Erasmus (Alive Books, 1996)
The Food Connection: The Right Food at the Right Time by Sam Graci (John Wiley & Sons, 2011)
The Food and Mood Handbook: Find Relief at Last from Depression, Anxiety, PMS, Cravings and Mood Swings by Amanda Greary (Thorsons, 2001)

How Your Mind can Heal your Body by David Hamilton (Hay House, 2008)

You Can Heal your Life by Louise L. Hay (Hay House UK, 2004)

Helping Ourselves: Guide to Traditional Chinese Food and Energetics by Daverick Leggett and Katherine Trenshaw (Meridian Press, 1994)

The Women's Guide to Homeopathy by Andrew Lockie and Nicola Geddes (Hamish Hamilton, 1992)

Encyclopaedia of Natural Medicine by Michael Murray and Joseph Pizzorno (Little, Brown and Company, 1998)

Women's Bodies, Women's Wisdom by Christiane Northrup (Piatkus, 2009)

Healing with Wholefoods by Paul Pitchford (North Atlantic Books, 1993)

Pain Relief Without Drugs: A Self-Help Guide for Chronic Pain and Trauma by Jan Sadler (Healing Arts Press, 2007)

Aromatherapy for Women: A Practical Guide to Essential Oils for Health and Beauty by Maggie Tisserand (Healing Arts Press, 1996)

Sugar and Your Health by Ray C. Wunderlich Jr (Good Health Publications, 1992)

ENVIRONMENTAL ISSUES

The Dioxin War: Truth and Lies About a Perfect Poison by Robert Allen (Pluto Press, 2004)

Our Stolen Future: Are We Threatening Our Fertility, Intelligence and Survival? – A Scientific Detective Story by Theo Colborn, Dianne Dumanoski and John Peterson Meyers (Abacus, 1997)

The Feminization of Nature: Our Future at Risk by D. Cadbury (Hamish Hamilton, 1997)

Healthy Beauty: Your Guide to Ingredients to Avoid and Products You Can Trust by Samuel S. Epstein and Randall Fitzgerald (Benbella Books, 2010)

E for Additives by Maurice Hanssen (Thorsons, 1987)

FERTILITY

Beautiful Babies, Fabulous Families, Wonderful World by Belinda Barnes (Foresight, 2010)

The Baby Making Bible: Simple Steps to Enhance your Fertility and Improve your Chances of Getting Pregnant by Emma Cannon (Rodale, 2010)

Fit for Fertility: Overcoming Infertility and Preparing for Pregnancy by Michael
   Dooley (Hodder & Stoughton, 2007)

COOKING

Wheatless Cooking: Including Gluten-free and Sugar-free Recipes by L. Coffey (Ten
   Speed Press, 2008)
Cooking Without Made Easy by Barbara Cousins (Thorsons, 2005)
Ottolenghi: The CookBook by Sami Tamimi and Yotam Ottolenghi (Ebury Press,
   2008)
Riverford Farm Cookbook by Guy Watson and Jane Baxter (Fourth Estate, 2008)
Grow Your Own Drugs: Easy Recipes for Natural Remedies and Beauty Treats by
   James Wong (Collins, 2010)

APPENDIX 3: FOOD INTOLERANCE CHECKER

- Are you extremely lethargic soon after eating?
- Do you often feel better if you don't eat?
- Did you have problems such as reflux or colic, glue ear, ear infections, eczema, asthma or recurrent tonsillitis when you were a child?
- Do you have repeated unexplained symptoms such as rashes, hives or eczema and often seem to be unwell?
- Do you suffer from unexplained sneezing?
- Do you suffer from excess mucus or catarrh in the throat, nose or sinuses?
- Do you regularly crave certain foods such as bread or cheese?
- Do you have dark circles under your eyes and a pale colour?
- Do you suffer from fluid retention (puffy face or weight that fluctuates regularly by two or more pounds from day to day)?
- Do you suffer from signs of an irritated bowel – wind, cramping, loose stools or constipation?

If you can answer yes to three or more of the above it is probable that you have an intolerance to a trigger food. There is a lot of cross-over between the symptoms of candida and food intolerances. This is because they are both caused by a weakened immune system or a less-than-optimal digestive environment. An overgrowth of candida will more often than not trigger food intolerances if left untreated.

The elimination diet is regarded by many practitioners of nutritional medicine as the most accurate way to identify the food you may be intolerant to. Suspect food will then need to be removed, ideally for three months, and reintroduced slowly to check if the body is still responding. During this period it is important to support and heal the digestive weaknesses. Following the Kickstart Cleanse and then the Nurture Diet as well as taking the recommended supplements will greatly improve your digestive and immune health, and reduce vulnerability to food intolerances. As food intolerances may indicate a low level of digestive enzymes, taking a digestive enzyme formula in combination with the recommended supplement programmes in Kickstart Cleanse and Nurture Diet would be beneficial.

It is important to do an elimination diet with the guidance of a nutritional therapist. Usually a food diary is used to work out suspect foods before an elimination diet as many of the problem foods tend to be key food groups such as:

• **Wheat** – this includes pasta, bread, pastries, pizzas, biscuits, cakes, many breakfast cereals, wheat crackers and battered food.
• **Dairy** – milk, cheese, yogurt. Most people can still tolerate small amounts of butter. See the section 'The Wrong Sort of Dairy' in Chapter 4. Consider reintroducing raw milk after three months.

Eliminate any particular food that you have *every day*, i.e. anything you feel you have too much of. This can include caffeine or apples for example. Variety is key in reducing your chances of developing food intolerances.

After three months, reintroduce one food you have eliminated every three days. For example on Monday reintroduce a little wheat, if there are no symptoms, reintroduce a little cheese on Wednesday and a coffee on Saturday. This will either identify that you have an intolerance to one of the foods still or that your intolerance has disappeared in the three-month period. Once they have been re-established into your diet remember not to go overboard, eat all your foods in moderation and try to keep your diet varied.

APPENDIX 4: HAVE I GOT A BLOOD SUGAR IMBALANCE?

- Do you frequently experience significant fluctuations in energy throughout the day?
- Do you feel that eating something sweet or having a stimulant such as coffee solves your energy low?
- Do you frequently feel tired or unable to concentrate in the mid-late afternoon?
- Despite a good eight hours of sleep do you still feel tired and groggy when you wake up?
- Do you often wake up hungry in the night or starving when you wake in the morning?
- Do you suffer from panic attacks and anxiety regularly?
- Do you skip meals regularly, such as breakfast?
- Do you crave sweet foods, alcohol or stimulants?
- If you go for a while without food do you feel irritable or shaky?
- Do you have a family history of type 2 diabetes?

If you can relate to three of more of the above you could have a blood sugar imbalance. The dietary changes outlined in this book and the recommended supplements are ideal for regaining blood sugar balance. It is also important to check with your GP to rule out the possibility of diabetes.

APPENDIX 5: HAVE I GOT CANDIDA OVERGROWTH?

- Do you suffer from intestinal bloating and wind, nausea, loose stools or constipation that is worse after eating sugar, yeast or refined carbohydrates?
- Do you have vaginal thrush, persistent itching or recurrent cystitis?
- Do you experience fuzzy-headedness, poor concentration and memory, fatigue, dizziness, mood swings, anxiety, headaches and/or irritability?
- Do you suffer from an itchy nose, oral thrush, post-nasal drip (drippy nose!), regular sore throats and/or bad breath?
- Do you have unexplained aches and pains in your joints e.g. not after exercise?
- Do you feel unwell in damp weather or mouldy, wet conditions?
- Do you react strongly to chemicals, perfumes, fumes, synthetics or tobacco smoke or become easily tipsy after a small amount of alcohol?
- Do you have multiple allergies and cravings for sweet or stodgy foods?
- Do you have a slow metabolism, low body temperature and easy weight gain?

If you can answer yes to four or more of these questions then you could have an overgrowth of candida. The dietary changes outlined in this book can really help. The recommended supplements will also work well to support the health of the gut and reduce candida overgrowth alongside taking a daily probiotic supplement. I highly recommend a high strength probiotic with natural anti-fungal ingredients. Take for a month. Your symptoms may feel as though they are getting worse as the probiotics start to work and the excess candida dies off. These usually subside after 10 days and you may then begin to experience the benefits such as increased energy, less bloating, and better digestion. If you do not start to feel better after 10 days, consult your nutritional therapist or medical practitioner.

Doing the Kickstart Cleanse is really important for you to realign the digestive environment if you have candida overgrowth. When you follow the Kickstart Cleanse avoid fruit for the entire 14 days. It would also be wise to avoid dried fruit and fruit juices as these and fresh fruit contain high amounts of natural fruit sugars called fructose. This is fine when candida overgrowth is not a problem, beneficial in fact, but can 'feed' the fungus if it is out of balance. After 14 days, introduce stewed fruit such as apple, pear or papaya but go gently. See how you fare and if you feel you are reacting to the natural sugar content, avoid for a whole month and then reintroduce in the same manner.

Avoid fermented products, yeast, vinegars and fungi such as mushrooms for a month. This includes any pickled foods, smoked foods (such as fish or smoked tofu), Marmite and Vegemite.

To ease symptoms of vaginal thrush, put a little live yogurt (about a teaspoon) onto a non-bleached panty liner overnight for a week. It sounds messy but the live yogurt will provide the good bacteria needed to reduce the fungal overgrowth. Or find a natural vaginal cream or suppository that contains *Lactobacillus acidophilus*; for example from the supplement company Biocare. Avoid using scented shower gels, soaps or enriched, perfumed loo roll. These upset the pH balance of the vaginal area and can exacerbate thrush.

APPENDIX 6: KEEPING CLEAN AND GREEN

Don't be lured into the marketing jargon using 'natural' or 'botanicals'. These can be misleading and imply the product does not contain any chemicals that can cause health concerns. Vet your skincare, cosmetics and household products for the following ingredients, which are particularly relevant to sufferers of endometriosis.

BEAUTY AND COSMETIC PRODUCTS
Parabens
(Alkyl parahydroxy benzoates, or butyl/methyl/ethyl/propyl/isobutyl paraben)

- A group of preservatives used in food and majority of cosmetics.
- Usually found as a cocktail of 5 different parabens: Methylparaben; Ethylparaben; Propylparaben; Butylparaben; Isoparaben
- This combination is found in nearly every product that is used on a daily basis: shampoos, shower gels, body lotions, facial creams, make up and baby products.
- Parabens can be absorbed rapidly through intact skin. After 8 hours of contact with the skin, 60% of Methylparaben, 40% of Ethylparaben and 20% of Propylparaben were found to cross the skin.[1]
- Parabens are oestrogenic. This oestrogenic effect increases oestrogen dominance and fuels the progression of endometriosis.
- They accumulate in fatty tissue and have been found in breast tumours.

Polychlorinated biphenyls (PCBs)
- Used in coolant, lubricants and insulation for electrical equipment as well as paints, dyes and rubber.
- PCBs accumulate in human fat through inhaling them from the air arround us.
- Found in rivers and lakes, these toxins weaken the immune system, damage neurological development, and behave like oestrogen in the body by mimicking the shape of the real hormone and 'docking' into oestrogen receptors, increasing oestrogenic activity in the body.

Bisphenol A
- A compound found in some plastics.
- It can leach into foods and the environment.

- It produces oestrogen-like effects making it a contributing factor to immune suppression and some cancers.

Phthalates

(Dibutyl (DBP), di(2-ethylhexyl) (DEHP), di-ethyl phthalate (DEP), butyl benzyl phthalate (BBP))

- A group of chemicals used as plasticisers in products such as nail polishes (to reduce cracking by making them less brittle) and hair sprays and as solvents and perfume fixatives in various other products.
- Dibutyl phthalate (DBP) and di(2-ethylhexyl) phthalate (DEHP), butyl benzyl phthalate (BBP or BzBP) are the most commonly used.
- Phythalates have been related to hormonal activity with adverse effects on reproductive systems.

Triclosan

(5-chloro-2 (2,4-dichlorophenoxy)-phenol) or Trade name – Microban

- A chlorophenol used in products such as toothpaste, soaps and body washes.
- Like parabens they bioaccumulate in fatty tissue strengthening their toxic effects. Swedish research published in 2002 found high levels of Triclosan in 60% of human breast milk samples.
- Dioxins (linked to the development of endometriosis) are formed when it is manufactured, incinerated or exposed to sunlight.

Formaldehyde

- A common preservative, germicide; fungicide and disinfectant found in cosmetics and nail varnish as well as furnishings and fabrics.
- It has been associated with the development and progression of endometriosis and delayed conception.
- Formaldehyde has been classified as a human carcinogen (cancer-causing substance) by the International Agency for Research on Cancer and as a probable human carcinogen by the US Environmental Protection Agency.
- Formaldehyde is banned from use in certain applications and in the EU the maximum allowed concentration in finished products is 0.2%. Any product that contains 0.5% or above has to include a warning that it contains formaldehyde.

HOUSEHOLD PRODUCTS: HOW TO MAKE YOUR HOUSE GREEN AND SPARKLY

- **Basic cleaning ingredients** (get ready to use a lot of bicarbonate of soda!) Soap, water, bicarbonate of soda (baking soda), vinegar, lemon juice, salt and a hard scrubbing brush take care of most household cleaning needs. Bicarbonate of soda and corn starch are good carpet deodorisers. Salt is a mild disinfectant and can be used as scouring powder.
- **For blocked drains** Pour bicarbonate of soda down the drain until it fizzes followed by boiling water. Alternatively, pour a handful of salt down the drain, followed by a kettle of boiling water. Soda crystals can also be used according to the packaging instructions.
- **For carpets** Shake bicarbonate of soda or corn starch, leave for an hour and then vacuum.
- **Dishwashing powder** Use one part borax to one part bicarbonate of soda.
- **Floors** Clean wooden floors with linseed wash from one of the recommended brands.
- **Fridges** Use white wine vinegar, diluted in a little water and use to wash the inside of the fridge.
- **Glass cleaner** Use half white wine vinegar and half water. This also cleans tiles and counter tops.
- **Kettles** Descale with one part water and one part vinegar. Bring to boil, leave to cool and rinse thoroughly.
- **Silver** If you have a small job, the best silver polish is white toothpaste. Dab some on your finger, and rub into the tarnish. For bigger pieces, use bicarbonate of soda and a clean, damp sponge. Make a paste of bicarbonate of soda and water. Scoop the paste on to the sponge, and rub the paste into the silver. Rinse with hot water and polish dry with a soft, clean cloth. For badly tarnished silver, leave the bicarbonate of soda paste on the silver for an hour or so, before cleaning off with the help of a sponge and hot water.
- **Toilets** Clean with vinegar or vinegar-based commercial solutions. Disinfect with borax.

REFERENCES

CHAPTER 1

1. Hassan, H.M., 1976, 'Incidence of endometriosis in diagnostic laparoscopy', *Journal Reproductive Medicine*, 16, 135.

2. Kolberg, R., 1997, 'NEWS: Endometriosis enigma: Do the cells themselves hold the crucial clues?', *Journal of NIH Research*, 9, 23–5.

3. http://www.google.co.uk/imgres?imgurl=http://assets.treesd.com/images/healthtree/articles/imgIOEsymptoms.jpg&imgrefurl=http://www.healthtree.com/articles/endometriosis/symptoms/&usg=__NZLrsJaV2sewIdNfsd5f3H1Dwug=&h=338&w=282&sz=17&hl=en&start=43&zoom=1&tbnid=t6YRmMIGLdVDrM:&tbnh=148&tbnw=127&ei=MQSvTfaAO5OxhQe59fTfAw&prev=/search%3Fq%3Dendometriosis%2Bchocolate%2Bcysts%26um%3D1%26hl%3Den%26client%3Dsafari%26sa%3DN%26rls%3Den%26biw%3D1597%26bih%3D1102%26tbm%3Disch0%2C949&um=1&itbs=1&iact=rc&dur=518&oei=nAOvTfe7EoK6hAfvn5HeAw&page=2&ndsp=43&ved=1t:429,r:10,s:43&tx=35&ty=86&biw=1597&bih=1102

4. http://www.google.co.uk/imgres?imgurl=http://www.acfs2000.com/assets/images/surgery_services/diagnostic_laparoscopy_1.jpg&imgrefurl=http://www.acfs2000.com/surgery_services/diagnostic-laparoscopy.html&usg=__H-LrINF8R47dZiiPAPMLrmDd894=&h=239&w=450&sz=125&hl=en&start=133&zoom=1&tbnid=6HsYXbMt-iG4KM:&tbnh=104&tbnw=196&ei=uQWvTYPYLYabhQeUosndAw&prev=/search%3Fq%3Dendometriosis%2Bchocolate%2Bcysts%26um%3D1%26hl%3Den%26client%3Dsafari%26sa%3DN%26rls%3Den%26biw%3D1597%26bih%3D1102%26tbm%3Disch0%2C3062&um=1&itbs=1&iact=hc&vpx=1097&vpy=681&d

5. DiZerega, G.S. *et al.*,1980, 'Endometriosis: Role of ovarian steroids in initiation, maintenance and suppression', *Fertility and Sterility*, 33, 649.

6. Lamb, K. *et al.*,1986, 'Family Traits analysis: A case-control study of 43 women with endometriosis and their best friends', *American Journal of Obstetrics & Gynecolology*, 154, 596.

7. Zondervan, K.T. *et al.*, 2001, 'The genetic basis of endometriosis', *Current Opinion in Obstetrics and Gynecology*, 13, 309–314.

8. Ridley, J.H., 1968, 'A review of facts and fancies', *Obstetrical & Gynecological Survey*, 23,1.

9. O'Connor, D.T., 'Endometriosis'. In: Singer A.J.J., ed. Current reviews in *Obstetrics and Gynaecology*. Vol. 12. Edinburgh, Scotland: Churchill Livingstone, 1987; 1–154.

10. Cramer, D.W. *et al.*,1986, 'The relation of endometriosis characteristics, smoking and exercise', *Journal of the American Medical Association*, 255, 1904.

11. Sutton, C., Jones, K. and Adamson, G. D., *Modern Management of Endometriosis* (Taylor & Francis, 2006)

12. Sampson J.A., 1925, 'Heterotropic or misplaced endometrial tissue', *American Journal of Obstetrics & Gynecology*, 10, 649.

13. Ayers, J.W.T. and Friendenstab, A.P., 1985, 'Uterotubal hypotonia associated with pelvic endometriosis', *The American Fertility Society*, 131, 26.

14. Sutton, C., Jones, K. and Adamson, G. D., *Modern Management of Endometriosis* (Taylor & Francis, 2006)

15. Lebovic, D.I. *et al.*, 2001, 'Immunobiology of endometriosis', *Fertility and Sterility*, 75 (1),1–10.

16. Thomas, Eric and Rock, John, *Modern Approaches to Endometriosis* (Kluwer Academic, 1991)

17. Koninckx, P.R. *et al.*,1994, 'Dioxin pollution and endometriosis in Belgium', *Human Reproduction*, 9,1001–2.

18. Research Registry of the Endometriosis Association

19. Endometriosis UK 2010 Survey

20. Research Registry of the Endometriosis Association

21. US EPA (1985) *Health Assessment for polychlorinated dibenzo-p-dioxins*. Office of Health and Environmental Assessment, EPA/600-8-84/014f.

22. Olive, D.L. *et al.*, 1985, 'Expectant management of hydrotubation in the treatment of endometriosis associated infertility', *Fertility and Sterility*, 44, 35–9.

23. Sutton, C.J.G. and Hill, D., 1990, 'Laser Laporoscopy in the treatment of endometriosis. A five year study', *British Journal of Obstetrics and Gynaecology*, 97, 181–5.

24 Sutton C.J.G. and Ewen, S.P., 'Abstract to the International Society of Gynaecological Endoscopy Meeting, Washington, DC', 1992: 73.

25. Bruner-Tran, K. *et al.*,1999, 'The potential role of environmental toxins in the pathophysiology of endometriosis', *Gynaecological & Obstetric Investigation*, Supplement, 45–56.

26. Bowman, R.E. *et al.*, 1989, 'Chronic Dietary Intake of 2,3,7,8-tetrachlorodibenzo-p-dioxin', *Fertility and Sterility*, 84(1), 67–74.

27. Sutton, C., Jones, K. and Adamson, G. David, *Modern Management of Endometriosis* (Taylor & Francis, 2006), p.286.

28. Research Registry of the Endometriosis Association

29. Nyholt, Dale, R. *et al.*, 2009, 'Common Genetic Influences Underlie Comorbidity of Migraine and Endometriosis', *Genetic Epidemiology*, 33(2), 105–113.

30. Ferrero, S. *et al.*, 2004, 'Increased frequency of migraine among women with endometriosis', *Human Reproduction*, 19(12), 2927–32.

31. Sutton, C.J.G. *et al.*,1994, 'Prospective, randomised, double-blind, controlled trial of laser laparoscopy in the treatment of pelvic pain associated with minimal, mild and moderate endometriosis', *Fertility and Sterility*, 62, 696–700.

32. Sutton, C.J.G. and Hill, D., 1990, 'Laser laporoscopy in the treatment of endometriosis. A five year study', *British Journal of Obstetrics and Gynaecology*, 97, 181–5.

33. Olive, D.L. *et al.*, 1985, 'Expectant management of hydrotubation in the treatment of endometriosis associated infertility', *Fertility and Sterility*, 44, 35–9.

34. Tepaske, R. *et al.*, 2001, 'Effect of preoperative oral immune-enhancing nutritional supplement on patients at high risk of infection after cardiac surgery: a randomised placebo-controlled trial', *Lancet*, 358, 696–701.

35. Nakamura, K. *et al.*, 2005, 'Influence of preoperative administration of omega-3 fatty acid-enriched supplement on inflammatory and immune responses in patients undergoing major surgery for cancer', *Nutrition*, 21(6), 639–49.

36. Figueira, P.G. *et al.*, 2011, 'Stem cells in endometrium and their role in the pathogenesis of endometriosis', *Annals of the New York Academy of Sciences*, 1221,10–7.

37. Du, H., and Taylor, H.S., 2007, 'Contribution of bone marrow-derived stem cells to endometrium and endometriosis', *Stem Cells*, 25(8), 2082–6. Epub 2007, Apr 26.

CHAPTER 2

1. Ehdin, Suzannah, *The Self-Healing Human* (Holistic Wellness Publication, 2003)
2. Leyland, N. *et al.*, 2010, 'Endometriosis: diagnosis and management', *Journal of Obstetrics and Gynaecology Canada* (SCOG), 32, S1–32.
3. Sesti, F. *et al.*, 2007, 'Hormonal suppression treatment or dietary therapy versus placebo in the control of painful symptoms after conservative surgery for endometriosis stage III-IV. A randomized comparative trial', *Fertility and Sterility*, 88(6),1541–7. Epub 2007, Apr 16.
4. National Diet and Nutrition Survey 2010
5. Mason, P. and Ruxton, C.H.S., 'Towards a Healthier Britain', commissioned by The Proprietary Association of Great Britain (PAGB), the UK trade association for manufacturers of branded over-the-counter (OTC) medicines and food supplements. Available at: http://www.pagb.co.uk/publications/pdfs/towardsahealthierbritain2010.pdf
6. The Soil Association 2011
7. Gearhardt, A.N., *et al.*, 2011, 'Can food be addictive? Public health and policy implications', *Addiction*, 106(7),1208–12 (doi: 10.1111/j.1360-0443.2010.03301.x). Epub 2011, Feb 14.
8. Avena, N.M. *et al.*, 2008, 'Evidence for sugar addiction: behavioral and neurochemical effects of intermittent, excessive sugar intake', *Neuroscience and Biobehavioral Reviews*, 32, 1, 20–39. Epub 2007, May 18.
9. Hoehn, S.K. *et al.*, 1979, 'Complex versus simple carbohydrates and mammary tumors in mice', *Nutrition and Cancer*, 1, 3, 27.
10. Santisteban, G.A. *et al*, 1985, 'Glycemic modulation of tumor tolerance in a mouse model of breast cancer', *Biochemical and Biophysical Research Communications*, 132(3), 1174–9.
11. Seeley, S., 1983, 'Diet and breast cancer: The possible connection with sugar consumption', *Medical Hypotheses*, 11, 3, 319–27.
12. Dmowski, W.P. *et al.*, 1994, 'The role of cell-mediated immunity in pathogenesis of endometriosis', *Acta Obstetricia et Gynecologica Scandinavia Supplement*, 159, 7–14.
13. Thomas, Eric and Rock, John, *Modern Approaches to Endometriosis* (Kluwer Academic Publishers, 1991), p.97.

14. Sinaii N. *et al.*, 2002, 'High rates of auto-immune and endocrine disorders, fibromyalgia, chronic fatigue syndrome and atopic disease among women with endometriosis: a survey analysis', *Human Reproduction*, 17, 10, 2715–2724.

15. Dmowski, W.P. *et al.*, 'The Role of cell-mediated immunity in pathogenesis of endometriosis', 1994, *Acta Obstetricia et Gynecologica Scandinavia Supplement*, 159, 7–14.

16. Goldin, B.R. and Gorsbach, S.L., 1984, 'The effect of milk and lactobacillus feeding on human intestinal bacterial enzyme activity', *The American Journal of Clinical Nutrition*, 39, 756–761.

17. Thomas, Eric and Rock John, *Modern Approaches to Endometriosis* (Kluwer Academic Publishers, 1991), p.97.

18. Mamdouh, H.M. *et al.*, 2011, 'Epidemiologic determinants of endometriosis among Egyptian women: A hospital-based case-control study', *The Journal of the Egyptian Public Health Association*, 86, 1–2, 21–6.

19. Friends of the Earth press briefing for Safer Chemicals Campaign 'Chemicals and Health'.

20. Nayyar, T. *et al.*, 2007, 'Developmental exposure of mice to TCDD elicits a similar uterine phenotype in adult animals as observed in women with endometriosis', *Reproductive Toxicology*, 23, 3, 326–36.

21. Rier, S.E. *et al.*, 1993, 'Endometriosis in rhesus monkeys following chronic exposure to 2,3,7,8-tetrachlorodibenzo-p-dioxin', *Fundamental and Applied Toxicology*, 21, 433–441.

22. Bruner-Tran, K.L. *et al.*, 2008, 'Dioxin may promote inflammation-related development of endometriosis', *Fertility and Sterility*, 89, 5, 1287–98. Epub 2008, Apr 18.

23. Bruner-Tran, K. *et al.*, 1999, 'The potential role of environmental toxins in the pathophysiology of endometriosis', *Gynaecological & Obstetric Investigation*, Supplement, 45–56.

24. Bruner-Tran, K.L. *et al.*, 2010, 'Dioxin and endometrial progesterone resistance', *Seminars in Reproductive Medicine*, 28, 1, 59–68. Epub 2010, Jan 26.

25. Holsapple, M.P. *et al.*, 1991, 'A review of two, three, seven, eight – tetrachlorodibenzo-P-dioxin-induced changes in immuno competene', *Toxicology*, 69, 219–255.

26. Bruner-Tran, K.L. *et al.*, 2008, 'Dioxin may promote inflammation-related development of endometriosis', *Fertility and Sterility*, 89, 5, 1287–98. Epub 2008, Apr 18.
27. Rier, S. and Foster, W., 2002, 'Forum: environmental dioxins and endometriosis', *Toxicological Sciences*, 70,161–170.
28. Birnbaum, L.S. and Cummings, A.M., 2002, 'Dioxins and Endometriosis: A Plausible Hypothesis', *Environmental Health Persepctives*, 110, 1, 15–21.
29. US EPA, 1994, 'Risk characterisation of dioxin and related compounds – Draft Dioxin Reassessment', Washington DC Bureau of National Affairs.
30. WHO, 'Level of PCBs PCDDs and PCDFs in breast milk', WHO Environmental Health Series, 1989.
31. Konickx, P.R. *et al.*, 1994, 'Dioxin Pollution and endometriosis in Belgium', *Human Reproduction*, 9, 1001–1002.
32. Bailey, M.T. and Coe, C.L., 2002, 'Endometriosis is associated with an altered profile of intestinal microflora in female rhesus moneys', *Human Reproduction*, 17, 7, 1704–1708.
33. Colborn, Theo, *Our Stolen Future: Are We Threatening Our Fertility, Intelligence, and Survival? A Scientific Detective Story* (Plume Books, 1997)
34. Ballweg, M.L. and the Endometriosis Association, *Endometriosis: The Complete Reference for Taking Charge of Your Health* (McGraw-Hill Professional, 2003)
35. U.S. EPA, 1979, 'EPA's Final PCB ban rule: 100 questions & answers to help you meet these requirements', Washington, DC, Office of Toxic Substances TS-799.
36. Whitlock, J.P., 1990, 'Genetic and molecular aspects of 2,3,7,8-tetrachlorodibenzo-p-dioxin action', *Annual Review of Pharmacology*, 30, 251–277.
37. Pulim, H.J. *et al.*, 1993, 'Effects of dioxins on thyroid function in newborn babies', *Lancet*, 339, 1303.
38. WomenLivingNaturally.com
39. Van Voorhis, B. J. *et al.*, 1996, 'The effects of smoking on ovarian function and fertility during assisted reproductive cycles', *Obstetrics & Gynecology*, 88, 5, 785–91.
40. Thorp, V.J.J., 1980, 'Effect of oral contraceptive agents on vitamin and mineral requirements', *Journal of the American Dietetic Association*, 76, 6, 581–4.

41. Ebadi, M. *et al.*, 1982, 'Drug-pyridoxal phosphate interactions', *Quarterly Review of Drug Metabolism Drug Interactions*, 4, 4, 289–331.

42. Webb, J.L., 1980, 'Nutritional effects of oral contraceptive use: A review', *The Journal of Reproductive Medicine*, 25, 4, 150–6.

43. British Medical Association, *Official Guide to Medicines and Drugs* (Dorling Kindersley, 2007)

44. White, E. *et al.*, 1994, 'Breast cancer among young US women in relation to oral contraceptive use'. *Journal of the National Cancer Institute.*, 86, 7, 505–14.

45. Brinton, L.A. *et al.*, 1995, 'Oral contraceptives and breast cancer risk among younger women', *Journal of the National Cancer Institute*, 87, 11, 827–35.

46. Olsson, H. *et al.*, 1991, 'Early oral contraceptive use and premenopausal breast cancer – A review of studies performed in southern Sweden', *Journal of Cancer Detection and Prevention*, 15, 4, 265–71.

47. Darbe, P.D., 2005, 'Aluminium, antiperspirants and breast cancer', *Journal of Inorganic Biochemistry*, 99, 9, 1912–9.

48. Gerhard, I. and Runnebaum, B., 1992, 'The limits of hormone substitution in pollutant exposure and fertility disorders', *Zentralbl Gynakol*, 114, 12, 593–602.

CHAPTER 3

1. Associate Parliamentary Food and Health Forum, 2008, 'The links between diet and Behaviour: The influence of nutrition on mental health'.

2. Soffritti, M. *et al.*, 2005, 'Aspartame induces lymphomas and leukaemias in rats', *European Journal of Oncology*, 10, 2, 107–116.

3. Lim, U. *et al.*, 2006, 'Consumption of aspartame-containing beverages and incidence of hematopoietic and brain malignancies', *Cancer Epidemiology, Biomarkers and Prevention*, 15, 9, 1654–1659.

4. Mier-Cabrera, J. *et al.*, 2008, 'Effect of vitamins C and E supplementation on peripheral oxidative stress markers and pregnancy rate in women with endometriosis', *International Journal of Gynecology and Obstetrics*, 100, 3, 252–6. Epub 2007, Nov 19.

5. Hay, William Howard, *Health Via Food* (Harrap, 1934)

6. Agarwal, A. *et al.*, 2005, 'Role of oxidative stress in female reproduction', *Reproductive Biology and Endocrinology*, 14, 3, 28.

7. Fugh-Berman, A. and Kronenberg, F., 2003, 'Complementary and alternative medicine (CAM) in reproductive-age women: A review of randomized controlled trials', *Reproductive Toxicology*, 17, 2, 137–52.

8. Fugh-Berman, A. and Kronenberg, F., 2003, 'Complementary and alternative medicine (CAM) in reproductive-age women: A review of randomized controlled trials', *Reproductive Toxicology*, 17, 2, 137–52.

9. Linos, E. *et al.*, 2010, 'Adolescent diet in relation to breast cancer risk among premenopausal women', *Cancer Epidemiology, Biomarkers & Prevention*, 19, 3, 689–96. Epub 2010, Mar 3.

10. Parazzini, F. *et al.*, 2004, 'Selected food intake and risk of endometriosis', *Human Reproduction*, 19, 8.

11. Grodstein, F. *et al.*, 1993, 'Relation of female infertility to consumption of caffeinated beverages', *American Journal of Epidemiology*, 137, 1353–60.

12. Lamb, K. and Nichols, T. R., 1986, 'Endometriosis: A comparison of associated disease histories', *American Journal of Preventative Medicine*, 2, 6, 324–9.

13. Shepperson Mills, Dian and Vernon, Michael, *Endometriosis: A key to healing and fertility through nutrition* (Thorsons, 2002)

CHAPTER 4

1. The Lancet Oncology: Special Release, 2011, 'International Agency Research on Cancer (IARC) classifies radiofrequency electromagnetic fields (including those caused by mobile phones) as possibly carcinogenic to humans'.

2. Li, D.K. *et al.*, 'A population based prospective cohort study of personal exposure to magnetic fields during pregnancy and the risk of miscarriage', *Epidemiology*, 13, 1, 9–20.

3. Röösli, M., 2008, 'Radiofrequency electromagnetic field exposure and non-specific symptoms of ill health: a systematic review', *International Journal of Environmental Research and Public Health*, 2, 277–87. Epub 2008, Mar 21.

4. Li, D.K. *et al.*, 'A population based prospective cohort study of personal exposure to magnetic fields during pregnancy and the risk of miscarriage', *Epidemiology*, 13, 1, 9–20.

5. Ehdin, Susanna, *The Self-Healing Human* (Holistic Wellness Publishers, 2003)

6. Waye, J.D., 1973, 'A short account of Chinese medicine', *Theories and philosophies of medicine*, compiled by Department of Philosophy of Medicine and Science (Tughlaqabad, New Delhi 62: Institute of History of Medicine and Medical Research).
7. US Food and Drug Administration Report, 1999, 'Tampons, Asbestos, Dioxins and Toxic Shock Syndrome'.
8. US EPA, 1985, 'Health assessment document for polychlorinated dibenzo-p-dioxins', Office of Health and Environmental Assessment, EPA/600-8-84/01 4f.
9. DeVito, M.J. and Schecter A., 2002, 'Exposure assessment to dioxins from the use of tampons and diapers', *Environmental Health Perspectives*, 110, 23–28.
10. Nassar S., 2003, 'Tampon Safety', National Centre for Policy Research (CPR) for Women and Families.
11. Kliman, Dr Harvey, *Gynecologic and Obstetrical Investigation* (June, 2002)
12. Ehdin, Susanna, *The Self-Healing Human* (Holistic Wellness Publishers, 2003)
13. Grohmann, U. *et al.*, 2003, 'Tolerance, DC's and tryptophan; much ado about IDO', *Trends in Immunology*, 24, 5, 242–248.
14. Mellor, A.L. and Munn, D.H., 2004, 'IDO expression by dendritic cells: Tolerance and tryptophan catabolism', *Nature Reviews Immunology*, 4, 10, 762–774.
15. Sharma, M.D. *et al.*, 2007, 'Plasmacytoid dendritic cells from mouse tumor-draining lymph nodes directly activate mature Tregs via indoleamine 2,3-dioxygenase, *The Journal of Clinical Investigation*, 117, 9, 2570–2582.
16. Facchinetti, F. *et al.*, 1983, 'Oestodial/progesterone imbalance and the premenstrual syndrome', *Lancet*, 2, 1302.
17. Ehdin, Susanna, *The Self-Healing Human* (Holistic Wellness Publishers, 2003)
18. Mills, D., 1992, 'Endometriosis: Possible nutritional strategies', *Lamberts Nutr Bull*, 2, 1–12.
19. G.E. Abraham, 'Primary Dysmennorhoea', *Clinical Obstetrics and Gynaecology*, 21, 1, 139–45.
20. Fugh-Berman, A. and Kronenberg, F., 2003, 'Complementary and alternative medicine (CAM) in reproductive-age women: A review of randomized controlled trials', *Reproductive Toxicology*, 17, 2, 137–52.

21. Ludwig, H., 1996, 'Dysmenorrhea', *Ther Umsch*, 53, 6, 431–41.

22. Zahradnik, H.P. and Breckwoldt, M., 1988, 'Drug therapy of dysmenorrhea', *Gynakologie und Geburtshilfe*, 21, 1, 58–62.

23. Campos Petean, C. *et al.*, 2008, 'Lipid peroxidation and vitamin E in serum and follicular fluid of infertile women with peritoneal endometriosis submitted to controlled ovarian hyperstimulation: A pilot study', *Fertility and Sterility*, 90, 6, 2080–5. Epub 2008, Feb 4.

24. Agarwal, A. *et al.*, 2005, 'Role of oxidative stress in female reproduction', *Reproductive Biology and Endocrinology*, 14, 3, 28.

25. Butler, E. B. and McKnight, E., 1995, 'Vitamin E in the treatment of primary dysmenorrhoea', *Lancet*, 268, 6869, 844–7.

26. Butler, E. B. and McKnight, E., 1995, 'Vitamin E in the treatment of primary dysmenorrhoea', *Lancet*, 268, 6869, 844–7.

27. Mier-Cabrera, J. *et al.*, 2008, 'Effect of vitamins C and E supplementation on peripheral oxidative stress markers and pregnancy rate in women with endometriosis', *International Journal of Gynecology and Obstetrics*, 100, 3, 252–6. Epub 2007, Nov 19.

28. Agarwal, A. *et al.*, 2005, 'Role of oxidative stress in female reproduction', *Reproductive Biology and Endocrinology*, 14, 3, 28.

29. Mathias, J.R. *et al.*, 1998, 'Relation of endomteriosis and neuromuscular disease of the gastrointestinal tract; new insights', *Fertility and Sterility*, 70, 81–7.

30. Kohama, T. *et al.*, 2007, 'Effect of French maritime pine bark extract on endometriosis as compared with leuprorelin acetate', *Reproductive Medicine*, 52, 8, 703–8.

31. Fugh-Berman, A. and Kronenberg, F., 2003, 'Complementary and alternative medicine (CAM) in reproductive-age women: A review of randomized controlled trials', *Reproductive Toxicology*, 17, 2, 137–52.

32. Mason, P. and Ruxton, C.H.S., 'Towards a Healthier Britain'. Commissioned by The Proprietary Association of Great Britain (PAGB), the UK trade association for manufacturers of branded over-the-counter (OTC) medicines and food supplements.

33. Wieser, F. *et al.*, 2007, 'Evolution of medical treatment for endometriosis: Back to the roots?', *Human Reproduction Update*, 13, 5, 487–99.

34. Jeong, S.J., *et al.*, 2011, 'Anti-angiogenic phytochemicals and medicinal herbs', *Phytotherapy Research*, 25, 1, 1–10.

35. Milewicz, A. *et al.*, 1993, 'Vitex agnus castus extract in the treatment of luteal phase defects due to latent hyperprolactinemia. Results of a randomized placebo-controlled double-blind study', *Arzneimittelforschung*, 43, 752–6.

36. Bartram, T., *Encyclopaedia of Herbal Medicine* (Grace Publishers, 1995)

37. Esfandiarei, M. *et al.*, 2011, 'Diosgenin modulates vascular smooth muscle cell function by regulating cell viability, migration, and calcium homeostasis', *Journal of Pharmacology and Experimental Therapeutics*, 336, 3, 925–39. Epub 2010, Dec 21.

38. Jung, D.H. *et al.*, 2010, 'Diosgenin inhibits macrophage-derived inflammatory mediators through downregulation of CK2, JNK, NF-kappaB and AP-1 activation', *International Journal of Immunopharmacology*, 10, 9, 1047–54. Epub 2010, Jun 11.

39. Weiser, F. *et al.*, 2007, 'Evolution of medical treatment for endometriosis: Back to the roots?' *Human Reproduction Update*, 13, 5, 487–499.

40. Eagon, P.K. *et al.*, 2000, 'Medicinal herbs: Modulation of estrogen action', Era of Hope Mtg, Dept Defense; Breast Cancer Res Prog, Atlanta, GA, Jun 8–11.

41. Nemeth, E. and Bernath J., 2008, 'Biological activities of yarrow species (*Achillea spp.*)', *Current Pharmaceutical Design*, 14, 29, 3151–67.

42. Groom, S.N. *et al.*, 2007, 'The potency of immunomodulatory herbs may be primarily dependent upon macrophage activation', *Journal of Medicinal Food*, 10, 1, 73–9.

43. Zakay-Rones, Z. *et al.*, 2004, 'Randomized study of the efficacy and safety of oral elderberry extract in the treatment of influenza A and B virus infections', *Journal of International Medical Research*, 32, 132–40.

44. Zakay-Rones, Z. *et al.*, 1995, 'Inhibition of several strains of influenza virus in vitro and reduction of symptoms by an elderberry extract (*Sambucus nigra L.*) during an outbreak of influenza B Panama', *Journal of Alternative and Complementary Medicine*, 1, 361–9.

45. Harrer, G. *et al.*, 1999, 'Comparison of equivalence between the St John's wort extract LoHyp-57 and Fluoxetine', *Arzneimittelforschung*, 49, 289–96.

46. Schrader, E., 2000, 'Equivalence of St. John'swort extract (Ze 117) and

Fluoxetine: A randomized, controlled study in mild-moderate depression', *International Clinical Psychopharmacology*, 15, 61–8.

47. Darbinyan, G., Aslanyan, G. and Amroyan, E., 2007, 'Clinical trial of Rhodiola rosea L. extract SHR-5 in the treatment of mild to moderate depression', *Nordic Journal of Psychiatry*, 61, 343–8.

48. Spasov, A.A. *et al.*, 2000, 'A double-blind, placebo-controlled pilot study of the stimulating and adaptogenic effect of Rhodiola rosea SHR-5 extract on the fatigue of students caused by stress during an examination period with a repeated low-dose regimen', *Phytomedicine*, 7, 85–89.

49. Bystritsky, A. *et al.*, 2008, 'A pilot study of Rhodiola rosea (Rhodax) for generalized anxiety disorder (GAD)', *Journal of Alternative and Complementary Medicine*, 14, 175–80.

50. Burks-Wicks, C., *et al.*, 2005, 'A Western primer of Chinese herbal therapy in endometriosis and infertility', *Women's Health*, 1, 3, 447–63.

51. Qu, F. *et al.*, 2005, 'The effect of Chinese herbs on the cytokines of rats with endometriosis', *Journal of Alternative and Complementary Medicine*, 11, 4, 627–30.

52. Flower, A. *et al.*, 'Chinese herbal medicine for endometriosis', *Cochrane Database of Systematic Reviews*, 2009

53. Han, J.S., 2004, 'Acupuncture and endorphins', *Neuroscience Letters*, 361, 1–3, 258–61.

54. Xiang, D.F. *et al.*, 2011, 'Effect of abdominal acupuncture on pain of pelvic cavity in patients with endometriosis', *Zhongguo Zhen Jiu*, 31, 2, 113–6.

55. Lundeberg, T. and Lund, I., 2008, 'Is there a role for acupuncture in endometriosis pain, or "endometrialgia"?', *Acupuncture in Medicine*, 26, 2, 94–110.

56. Xiang, D. *et al.*, 2002, 'Ear acupuncture therapy for 37 cases of dysmenorrhea due to endometriosis', *Journal of Traditional Chinese Medicine*, 22, 4, 282–5.

57. Canon, Emma, *The Baby Making Bible* (Rodale, 2010)

CHAPTER 6
1. Soil Association Report, 'An inconvenient truth about food', 2008.

CHAPTER 8

1. Johnson, N.P. *et al.*, 2005, 'Tubal flushing for subfertility', *Cochrane Database of Systematic Reviews*, 2, CD003718.
2. Adamson, G.D. *et al.*, 1993,'Laparoscopic treatment: Is it better?', *Fertility and Sterility*, 59, 35–44.
3. Yap, C. *et al.*, 2004, 'Pre and post operative medical therapy for endometriosis surgery', *Cochrane Database of Systematic Reviews*, 3, CD003678.
4. Jones, K.D. and Sutton, C.J.G., 2002, 'Pregnancy rates following ablative laparoscopic surgery for endometriomas', *Human Reproduction*, 17, 782–785.
5. Jacobson, T.Z. *et al.*, 2002, 'Laparoscopic surgery for subfertility associated with endometriosis', *Cochrane Database of Systematic Reviews*, 4, CD001398.
6. Thomas, E. and Rock, J., *Modern Approaches to Endometriosis* (Kluwer Academic Publishers, 1991), p119.
7. Thomas, Eric and Rock, John, *Modern Approaches to Endometriosis* (Kluwer Academic Publishers, 1991), p124.
8. Wiegand, K.C. *et al.*, 2010, 'ARID1A Mutations in endometriosis-associated ovarian carcinomas', *The New England Journal of Medicine*, 363, 16, 1532–1543.
9. Wiegand, K.C. *et al.*, 2010, 'ARID1A Mutations in endometriosis-associated ovarian carcinomas', *The New England Journal of Medicine*, 363, 16, 1532–1543.

APPENDIX 6: KEEPING CLEAN AND GREEN

1. Pedersen, S. I. *et al.*, 2007, 'In vitro skin permeation and retention of parabens from cosmetic formulations', *International Journal of Cosmetic Science*, 29, 5, 361–367.

INDEX

ACKNOWLEDGEMENTS

When I started this book I had no idea how *actually* writing it would need to involve so many people. Firstly I have to thank Charlie, Alfie and Ned for their tireless support and patience, giving me the space I needed to do this. I am, and will remain, indescribably grateful. To my dear ma for reading draft after draft, and for contributing her writing expertise along the way.

Thank you too to Clare Hulton and Kyle for believing that I could write this much needed book. And a special thanks to Vicky Orchard for her editorial support, her hawk eye for detail, and in fact all those at Kyle Books who helped with the process along the way.

I could not have done this without the help of experts in their field: Professor Chris Sutton, Michael McIntyre and expert and lovely friend, chef Louise Henkel.

To the Tigmi Hotel, Marrakech for providing its timeless, unquantifiable magic at a time of much needed rest. God given. And a thank you to Dick and his wife for their adaptor plug for my laptop whilst I was there!

And last but far from least to my patients. For trusting me with their health and working as a team during their journey; I learn from them every day.